Contagion

Contagion

Perspectives from Pre-Modern Societies

Edited by

Lawrence I. Conrad
and Dominik Wujastyk

Ashgate

Aldershot • Burlington USA • Singapore • Sydney

Published by

Ashgate Publishing Limited
Gower House
Croft Road, Aldershot
Hants GU11 3HR
England

Ashgate Publishing Company
131 Main Street
Burlington
Vermont 05401-5600
USA

Ashgate website: http://www.ashgate.com

British Library Cataloguing in Publication Data
Contagion: Perspectives from Pre-Modern Societies.
1. Communicable diseases–History. 2. Communicable diseases–Social aspects–History. 3. Medicine, Ancient.
I. Conrad, Lawrence I., 1949– II. Wujastyk, Dominik.
306. 4' 61' 0901

US Library of Congress Control Number: 00–104025

ISBN 0 7546 0258 3

This book is printed on acid free paper

Designed and typset with TEX at the Wellcome Institute for this History of Medicine.

Printed and bound by Athenaeum Press, Ltd.,
Gateshead, Tyne & Wear.

CONTENTS

PREFACE

The papers in this volume were originally presented at a conference on contagion in pre-modern societies held at the Wellcome Institute for the History of Medicine in 1993. Since then, the papers have been substantially revised for publication. A goal of that conference was to explore a key concept in medical history across the boundaries not only of time, but also of culture and language. This goal remains central to the present volume. Historians are, by definition, professionally concerned with negotiating the pathways of past time, to which medical historians must add a specifically medical insight. But all too often the apparent otherness of cultural and linguistic difference presents a barrier which is not negotiated, and many histories claiming generality in reality focus on small, bounded parts of the "western" world, and exclude relevant data which happens to be recorded in non-European languages. It is therefore a source of special satisfaction to be able to present this volume, in which the history of an important medical concept is genuinely chased down in all parts of the globe, and through sources produced in many classical and modern languages from both East and West. This effort has involved the collaboration of historians with exceptionally wide-ranging skills in languages and in cultural studies, and has been an enriching experience for all concerned with the preparation of this book.

It is the pleasant duty of the editors to acknowledge the assistance of Mohsina Somji in preparing the typescript of this volume. We would also like to thank Barbara Hird, registered indexer of the Society of Indexers, for preparing the index with such care and precision.

Introduction

'Contagion' – even today the word conjures fears of serious disease, of uncontrollable outbreaks of drug-resistant bacteria, of viruses like Ebola and HIV. Older terrors such as malaria, cholera, and even tuberculosis, are still extremely dangerous and continue to kill people in large numbers. The progress of the biomedical sciences is shadowed by the parallel process of adaptation and mutation amongst pathogens, so that the threat of new outbreaks of contagious disease remains a very present one. Popular treatments of contagion in fiction, printed and film, today attract mass audiences, as they have at least since the fourteenth century, when Boccaccio framed his *Decameron* as tales told while in refuge from a devastating plague, which he did not hesitate to describe in gory detail. The idea of contagion clearly retains the power to fascinate and terrify.

Contagious disease was an even greater threat to past generations of mankind all over the world. Diseases like bubonic plague, smallpox, syphilis, tuberculosis, cholera, and influenza, which are today preventable or treatable in varying degrees, killed adults and children in vast numbers. Although the biomedical sciences provide the dominant contemporary explanatory model for contagious disease, broadly speaking in terms of germ theory, there remains a certain cognitive dissonance in the minds of many people outside the medical establishment. When AIDS first emerged as a global health problem, there was no shortage of irrational voices claiming that the disease was a punishment for an immoral lifestyle. In some ways this echoed the theological debates which surrounded the discovery of smallpox vaccination at the end of the eighteenth century. At that time many opposed vaccination on the grounds that disease was a just punishment for sin. Today, popular beliefs about disease causation are by no means always closely aligned with the current medical orthodoxy. In early 1999, Glen Hoddle, coach of the England football team, was widely vilified in the press, and subsequently obliged to resign, for publicly stating his belief that disease and disability were attributable to *karma*, a view, moreover, proposed two thousand years ago in Indian medical texts (see p. 94 below). If there is such variation at the popular level in our explanatory models for disease today, we naturally expect to find varied and interesting explanations in the past as well.

Words and ideas

That certain diseases are readily transmitted from an ill person to a healthy one is something that one might expect that all pre-modern societies would have noticed and explained in some way. As several papers in this volume show, the phenomenon of contagion was recognised by society at large, and was especially clear to pastoralists and those charged with the care of animals, who did not need great epidemics to observe the spread of disease among their herds (158–60, 168–71). Both Chinese and Indian doctors posed the question of why many people should all fall prey to a single disease at a single time and place (5, 93). But for the modern historian one of the first questions to arise is, as Vivian Nutton puts it in the title of his paper in this volume, "did they have a word for it?" This is not a philological quibble, but raises the question of whether a given culture's thinking on contagion resulted in the emergence of specific terminology and vocabulary precisely expressing what it understood the process of 'contagion' to comprise.

In some cases such terminology clearly did exist. The Latin *contagio* and the Arabic *'adwā*, for example, encompass notions of touch, transmission, and transitiveness, and in medical contexts they appear in contexts of danger of proximity, pollution, and defilement. So in such cases the modern English translation "contagion" seems to be quite apt (138, 163–64). But already a problem arises, in that while pre-modern notions of 'contagion' often include the modern understanding of the idea, they are seldom limited to this sense. The terms *contagio* and *'adwā* were terms referring to a disease's transmissibility in general, and included transmission through heredity. In fact, it is clear from the studies in this volume that the modern epidemiological distinctions between contagion and infection remained unknown throughout the world until modern times (164). Even in the English language, the distinction has never been firm, outside the learned usage of medical professionals. The *Oxford English Dictionary*, in a passage which could almost be a translation from one of our early non-western, records that Trevisa wrote in 1398 of leprosy as a "contagyon" which was passed from parent to child as if by heredity. In 1603 Lodge defined contagion more precisely as "an evil qualitie in a bodie, communicated vnto an other by touch...". In the late eighteenth century, contagion could still be spoken of as being communicated through the air: the 1751 edition of Chambers' authoritative *Cyclopedia* claimed that "in other [diseases] the contagion is transmitted through the air to a great distance, by means of steams, or effluvia, expiring from the sick." Figurative use of the word was also common: Chaucer spoke in 1386 of the soul being troubled by the "contagion of my body", and in 1592, Junius referred in his commentary on *Revelations* to "the contagion of sin".

It is interesting to find that cultures with great literary traditions of medicine often did not have specific terms for contagion. Greek medicine, for example, lacked such a vocabulary; or at least, terms that could convey the notion of contagion very well, such as *epaphe* and *synanachrosis*, were never widely used (138–42). Similarly, as Das's discussion reveals, Sanskrit medical texts employ several terms whose possible technical meanings are hard, if not impossible, to distinguish from ordinary-language usage (55–69). Instead, one routinely finds that situations asserting the danger of proximity, for example, are described without recourse to any well-defined technical term for the principle under discussion.

Where specific terminology does exist, there are still other obstacles at a basic level. The Latin *contagio* may appear rather frequently, but nowhere in ancient Latin literature does an author discuss the process he has in mind when using this word (149), and in many cases it comprises a synonym for 'disease' and refers to the progression within the body—rather like putrefaction or 'colouring'—of some illness that had originated there (188–89, 191). It is therefore a great error to assume that when a Latin author uses it he is referring to the transmission of a disease entity, as almost any modern observer would do. Much material on the Arabic term *'adwā* is to hand, but from the discussion studied in this volume it is already clear that it had two rather different ranges of signification, one associated with spirits and the spread of disease through malevolent supernatural processes (165), and a second located squarely within formal humoral medicine and explained by the revival of this system in the wake of a vigorous translation movement that made many of the works of Galen available in Arabic (173–74). A similar ambivalence is visible in the Sanskrit texts studied by Das and Zysk, where the medieval commentators argue that some kinds of contagion are supernatural, while others are more closely involved with what we might today call natural phenomena (63–67, 91–92).

There are cases in which an implicit sense of contagion is borne by a word or phrase that does not always or usually have this meaning. A good example of this is the Hebrew *ṣāraʿat*, which is usually translated as leprosy, but can also refer to a 'contagious' fungal infestation (104). On the other hand, such implicit significations can quickly prove awkward to the modern researcher, as one can see in references to Muslims being "on their guard" against the blind and the lame, which implies a belief that not only illness, but also physical disability, can be transmitted to healthy individuals (166).

There is also the question of whether or not the principle being invoked is one of medical observation. In the Hebrew Old Testament, for example, it is stated that a man with a genito-urinary discharge must be isolated so long as the condition persists (99, 117–18). This has to do with canons of ritual purity rather than medical awareness of contagion, as is made clear in the passage itself, where God specifies that the measure is required so that "they should not defile (i.e. render ritually unclean) their camps in which I dwell" (115). Lieber's paper in fact highlights the extent to which *ṣāraʿat* was viewed as a problem brought on by sin (107 n. 28, 108, 111), or as a warning for lack of faith (111). For the Latin usage of *contagio* Nutton urges caution, since even in contexts where the term must by rendered as 'contagion', what was meant was not the transmission of a disease, but rather an emanation, an effluxion, a breath, a poison, a putrid effusion, an excrement, or a miasma, or in moral terms, a pollutant or contaminant (151–54). And for the Latin West Touati exposes a number of cases where a perception of contagion has erroneously been read into a medieval text concerning leprosy, based on the researcher's a priori expectations rather than what the passage actually says (183–85).

Social context

These last observations indicate how important the broader social and cultural context was in forming and shaping ideas of contagion.

Several of the studies in this volume demonstrate that demonology was an important and multi-cultural factor in shaping ideas of contagion. Belief in the role of demons and spirits of various kinds as bearers and agents of disease was very common, and this necessarily played an important role in perceptions of contagion. Traces of a very early concept of seizure by a demon may survive in the Old Testament accounts of *ṣāraʿat* (120–21). In Islam, the transmission of disease was often explained as the work of the *jinn* (165–67). The same was true of India where, from the second millennium BC, disease was commonly viewed as the work of demons (69–70, 85–86, 91–92). In China too, demonic influence was a standard theme in medicine and, as in India, children were seen as especially vulnerable to sudden illness, whether through demonic or adventitious attack. Cullen shows how the malevolent influence of the threatening stranger was thought to cause disease especially in children, through a kind of contagion, and Chang describes how the belief in a fetal toxin led directly to the development of the technique of smallpox variolation in the period of the Late Ming Dynasty (1368–1644).

In societies organised around the tenets of religion, ritual and religious law could dominate customary practice and thus sometimes contributed in major ways to thinking on contagion. Among the Israelites, *ṣāra'at* was usually conceived of in terms of ritual purity and religious law, and in a system in which the distinction between ritually clean and unclean was extremely important, contagious disease was of interest for the danger it posed of contamination (115-21). In Islamic society, the central problem posed by contagion was that it seemed to threaten the monotheistic doctrine of God as the author and orderer of all things. If serious and often fatal illness befell a healthy individual, this could only be by the will and permission of God, not by reason of exposure or proximity to someone else already ill with the disease. As Conrad's paper shows, using one case in which the issues are clearly articulated, concern about this problem eventually led Muslim scholars to reject contagion, at least in its animistic form (166–67). This then elevated contagion into an archetype for argument over larger theological issues of religious authority.

In India, by contrast, although the caste system was fundamentally a social expression of the purity–pollution gradient, these ritual concepts did not influence, and were apparently not influenced by, medical thinking. One would have thought that the caste concepts of ' touchable' and 'untouchable' (Skt. *spṛśya / aspṛśya*) would be natural candidates from which a theory of contagion might develop, but this was not the case. In general, Indian medical thought was carried out orthogonally to social and religious doctrine. The recommendations of medicine (*āyurveda*) were sometimes at odds with socio-religious mores (*dharma*), with little attempt being made to harmonize conflicting value systems except through the standard practices of atonement and penance after the fact.

It also emerges that formal medical thinking could itself impact upon perceptions of contagion in unexpected ways. The lack of any prominent contagion theory in Greek medical texts calls for explanation. For the classical Western humoral tradition, Nutton suggests that one reason—but not a sufficient one—may lie in the fact that such theory appeared mechanistic, which would have been unattractive to authors like Galen (156). For the Latin tradition of the medieval West, which was founded on the Greek (largely as a second remove, based on Arabic translations of Greek texts), Touati suggests that humoral theory itself may have had a negative impact on contagion theory, since the humoral system, especially with the doctrine of miasma in play, was already sufficient to explain the spread of disease and thus did not encourage the level of discussion that would have been required for contagion to rise to a prominent place in European humoral medical thinking; in any case, the accommodation of contagion as a major element in medical thinking would have required the postulation and acceptance of an abstract separation—wholly unlikely in humoral terms—between a disease entity and the individual carrying it (188–92). Conrad's ninth-century case study from an Islamic point of view illustrates quite clearly how useful miasma was as a tool in efforts to deny or limit contagion; the danger of proximity to or contact with an ill individual could easily be restated in terms of exposure to corruption in the air, thus sharply reducing the need to exploit the explanatory value of contagion theory to the extent that it might otherwise have been pursued (169–70).

Similarly, in both India and Greece, as Zysk describes (93–95), doctors analyzed the natural environment in a comparable manner, isolating the elements of air, water, land, and season as necessary and sufficient causative factors in epidemic disease. These notions were considered adequate to explain the simultaneous appearance of a particular disease amongst many different individuals in a community. Kuriyama convincingly argues that the relative obscurity of contagion theory in China is due to the fact that other factors were perceived as more critical, that doctors were overwhelmingly preoccupied by other 'more urgent' concerns (12). In particular, they too were concerned with counteracting the ubiquitous effects of the natural environment on their human patients. In China this environment was principally manifested through the effects of weather, which was seen as a prime etiological factor in disease.

There was also the matter of social constraints. As Nutton points out, a prominent doctrine of contagion might be expected to have certain practical consequences—exclusion of the ill and quarantine. But it was not within the power of the doctors or of municipal authorities to enforce either, and movement at any level in this direction would have required society to abandon that most sacred of moral duties, to care for one's kin and dependents (160–61).

It also emerges that authors could sometimes write differently for different audiences. The ninth-century polymath Ibn Qutayba, for example, was prepared to be very critical of contagion theory in contexts where it threatened the authority of sayings of the Prophet Muḥammad; outside this arena, however, it is clear that he was quite willing to accept, or at least to include in his books, material that implicitly embraced contagion (174–75).

As ideas of contagion emerged from a complex social and cultural matrix of related ideas, changes and developments in a culture would of course result in changes in the way in which contagion was viewed. A vivid example of this can be seen in how the Greek vocabulary of metaphor for contagion shifted when it passed into the hands of speakers of Latin or Arabic: the Greeks' metaphors of sharing and pollution become those of touching in Latin, and transference or transmission in Arabic (142, 163–64). A similar development can be seen in the perception of leprosy in Europe, where the emergence of a sharply negative attitude toward lepers and the danger of their proximity does not arise until the early decades of the thirteenth century. Even then its growth was at first slow and limited (192–98).

It is worth adding here that, as Chang has described, the practice of Chinese smallpox variolation arose in conjunction with a rational and plausible theoretical model of the disease and its aetiology, namely that of 'fetal toxin' (23–38). When the technique of variolation spread to other parts of the world, including India, Turkey, and Britain, its original rationale was left behind, and only the outer form of the method was transmitted. That this was effective, and gave mankind its first effective weapon against a terrible disease, is not in question. But it is interesting to see here an example of the quarrying of a foreign medical system for methods and medicines which are—in the process of transmission—divorced from their epistemological and social roots. What is taken is pure technique, or technology, but not the scientific justification for the technique. This reminds us of the issues surrounding 'green imperialism', raised once again in recent years connection with the granting of a USA patent to a process for preserving an extract from the Neem (*Azadirachta indica* A. Juss.), a tree whose medicinal properties have been known in India for millennia.

Overall, contagion must be viewed as a doctrine whose prominence in a given tradition depended upon a wide range of factors both medical and non-medical. The question to be asked is therefore not why the medical tradition of this or that people failed to notice or comment upon a doctrine that to modern sensibilities is obvious and not only relevant, but crucial, to any effective response to large-scale disease phenomena. Nor is it particularly illuminating to address the matter in terms of some postulated dichotomy—again the issue of arbitrary imposition of value based on the retrojection of modern thinking arises—between 'advanced' and 'primitive' peoples (182). Rather, what needs to be addressed is whether and how the range of relevant influences both from within medicine and from society at large served to encourage or discourage the formation, discussion, and widespread acceptance of contagion theory within the society in question.

Social reaction

How did society react to the presence in its midst of individuals suffering from contagious diseases? For example, a question we might ask is whether the fear of 'the threatening stranger' (*kewu*) as a source of poisonous *qi* caused tensions in the Chinese system of mutual hospitality. Cullen points out that the *kewu* was not necessarily as dominant a concept in medical practice as it was in medical textbooks (53–55), but it is highly likely to have been a widespread reality in folk medicine and common belief, as indeed similar fears about 'demon-infected' strangers were in India.

In many societies, religious ideology strongly determined such reactions. In a society in which contagious disease was perceived in terms of ritual purity and possible sinfulness, one afflicted with such a disease was subject to examination by a priest, who would decide on further measures (116–17). In medieval Islam the debate over contagion illustrates how central the defense or repudiation of the authority of Prophetic traditions—i.e., issues of dogmatics and theology—was to attitudes toward contagion (167–73).

Another reaction could be that of exclusion. In some cases, as among the ancient Israelites, lepers were excluded, at least for as long as they were ill (114, 127–28), and sometimes for fixed periods (121), though this was not regarded as a punishment. Readmission to society required rituals of purification. But in other cases this was not so. In early medieval Europe, for example, and contrary to the findings of much previous modern scholarship, lepers were not excluded from society and indeed seem to have enjoyed free association with the rest of the community (184–85, 188, 199–201).

Atonement rituals were required if one had been infected as a result of sin or religious shortcomings (117–18). Atonements (*prāyaścitta*) and penance vows (*vrata*) were very highly developed forms of religious and social expression in India, and were the normal recourse of those who had abrogated righteousness (*dharma*), thereby causing, for example, epidemics (93).

In some societies, the threat of contagion led directly to the institution of public health measures. Medieval Islam provides a valuable case of a society in which public health measures against contagion were clearly being implemented, while at the same time contagion theory was quite controversial (176–77). What this seems to indicate is that society was prepared to accommodate the subject in multiple contradictory registers, with contagion being critiqued and often denied in religious scholarship, while it was accepted as a matter of course in more practical secular spheres.

Methodological issues

It is important to note that there was a profoundly pluralistic outlook on contagion in the pre-modern world, not only between the various cultures and societies considered in this volume, but also within a given culture, and even within a specific corpus of material: for example, the *Huangdi neijing* in China, the works of the Hippocratics in Western antiquity, the *āyurvedic* corpus in India, or the opera of Ibn Qutayba in ninth-century Iraq. The peril of assuming uniformity over vast domains of time and space are of course well known, but are particularly acute for areas of research where evidence is thin on the ground and often difficult to interpret; Touati's contribution clearly highlights such difficulties in past scholarship.

This requires, in the first instance, a close examination of text and context, an effort to discover what the text means in terms of the social milieu from which it emerged. It is only in this way that research can avoid the pitfalls stressed by Das, Nutton and Touati: tendencies to read ancient and medieval texts as if they were, to borrow Nutton's metaphor, lectures prepared for presentation to the Royal Society of Medicine (151), and failure to take into account changes and development over time, as in the case of medieval Europe's reaction to leprosy (180, 198–99). Touati's paper is in fact a useful critique of the ways in which subtle but major methodological errors can lead scholarship far astray.

Equal care has to be taken not to underestimate the degree to which ancient ideas survive in contemporary times. In 1898, just one year after the Indian plague pandemic of 1896–97, one P. Murlidhar Sharma published in Bombay a tract called *Mahāmārī kā vivecana [An inquiry into plague]: origin of plague and its cure.* In Hindī and Sanskrit he presented for popular consumption a two-thousand year old account of the causes and treatment of plague which was completely at odds with the techniques which the British health and sanitary authorities had been applying. The firm distinctions between ancient and modern learning common in Western thinking, along with their judgemental implications concerning the progress of science, clearly become problematic in other cultural contexts in which medical texts written over a millennium ago are routinely printed as contributions to contemporary medicine, not as historical sources.

Another vital point is that of contextuality. Issues of context of course involve not only the material surrounding a given passage in the rest of the text to which it belongs, but also the broader range of literary and other evidence that may be relevant to one's investigation. As Touati so aptly puts it: "Medical writings are never autonomous" (201). It will be noted that papers in this volume draw upon such under-exploited materials as poetry, theology, dogmatics, and even within medical literature, veterinary tracts. The complexity of the task at hand, the loss of much of what had once been written, and the need to avoid—in so far as this is possible—reading the past in terms of the present, make it essential to base research on as broad a range of the extant source material as possible.

Perhaps a final point may be made concerning the difficulty of controlling source materials in the non-western traditions. The vastness of the evidence available in Asian medical traditions is remarkable. It may reasonably be said that material for Greek and Roman antiquity is now fairly well in hand, at least so far as research and reference tools and availability of good critical editions are concerned. The same can be said for Old Testament studies, which are also mature and well equipped with the aids required for detailed advanced research, and to a lesser extent the same is true of medieval Europe. But this does not necessarily hold the great non-Western cultures of ancient and medieval times. Basic reference works are often lacking or outdated. Many medical texts are still only known as entries in nineteenth-century manuscript catalogues. And the literary materials available for study are orders of magnitude more voluminous than those for Classical or Old Testament studies. Thus many of the papers presented here deal with specific cases or representative topics. In spite of these real challenges, the authors in this volume between them convey a vivid and engaging picture of human responses to contagious disease in past ages, full of culture-specific subtleties and unexpected inversions of meaning.

DOMINIK WUJASTYK
LAWRENCE I. CONRAD

Part I

CHINA

1

Epidemics, Weather, and Contagion in Traditional Chinese Medicine

Shigehisa Kuriyama

In the early decades of the third century devastating epidemics spread through China. "Each family knew the pain of death," testified the poet Cao Zhi (192–32), "and from each room came wails and cries of sorrow." Many blamed demons and gods, and sought to avert harm by hanging talismans on their portals. But Cao Zhi thought such people foolish. He noted that it was mostly the poor who died; and he traced the affliction to a disordering of the *yin* and the *yang*, a chaotic confusion of the cold and the hot.[1]

Why do hundreds, and thousands, and hundreds of thousands of people suddenly fall violently ill, and die, around the same time, with similar symptoms? What explains the swift, terrifying sweep of epidemics? It was an urgent question, and for much of Chinese history two kinds of answers held sway.

There was, on the one hand, the appeal to influences demonic and divine. Cao Zhi's skepticism notwithstanding, belief in malign powers was hardly confined to an ignorant populace. The *Shiming* dictionary (second century) glossed *yi*, epidemics, as *yi*, corvée, the harsh servitude from which there is no escape, and elaborated, "It refers to the corvée exacted by demons." Even Zheng Xuan, one of the most learned of Han dynasty scholars, taught that

The following abbreviations are used in this chapter:

WYLP: Zhejiang sheng zhongyi yanjiusuo. *Wenyilun pingzhu* (Beijing: Renmin weisheng chubanshe, 1977);
ZBYHL: *Zhubing yuanhou zonglun* (Taipei: Guoli zhongguo iyao yanjiusuo, 1964);
SKQS: *Wenyuange siku quanshu* (Taipei: Shangwu inshuguan);
YBQS: *Yibu quanshu* (Taipei: Yiwen inshuguan, 1977).

[1] Cao Zhi, "Shuo yiqi," in Zhao Yongwen ed., *Cao Zhi ji jiaozhu* (Beijing: Renmin wenxue chubanshe, 1984), 177. Cited in Kanô Yoshimitsu, *Chûgoku igaku no tanjô* (Tokyo: Tokyo daigaku shuppankai, 1987), 61.

the appearance of certain stars in the sky foretold the rampaging of pestilential demons(*ligui*).[2] Influential too was the cosmo-political interpretation, according to which epidemics, along with droughts and other catastrophes, were triggered by transgressions against the will of Heaven by the Emperor, the Son of Heaven. In 163, the Emperor Wendi himself acknowledged this as a possible cause of the disasters in his time—though he denied, in the same breath, any inkling of where he might have erred.[3]

Medical writings, on the other hand, echoed Cao Zhi's opinion. The *Shanghan lun* (*Treatise on cold-damage disorders*) attributed to Cao Zhi's contemporary, Zhang Ji, elaborated a comprehensive system of diagnosis and treatment based on the premise that winds, harsh cold, and the like commonly inflict serious, even mortal harm. Up into the nineteenth century, this premise remained at the heart of how most Chinese doctors explained epidemics. For over two thousand years, they traced the ravages of shared sickness to, above all, the impact of shared weather.

Chen Yan's (twelfth-century) views are telling. In a scheme cited approvingly by many after him, the Song dynasty physician parsed diseases into three types: those of internal origin, those of external origin, and those of origins neither inner nor outer. The first designated ailments arising from anger, or grief, joy, fear, love, hatred, shock; the second referred to sicknesses brought by wind and cold, heat, dryness, the damp; and into the third category fell all the afflictions due to all other causes—overeating, starvation, sexual dissipation, wolves and tigers, demons, parasites, poisons, broken limbs, the wounds of war. People fell ill, in short, for many different reasons, but two factors mattered most: the emotions and the weather. Weather was *the* external threat. All the other dangers in the surrounding world ranked only as miscellaneous concerns.

A synopsis of the traditional Chinese understanding of epidemics might reasonably stop here. Demons, heavenly displeasure, the attacks of wind and cold, and the emotional exhaustion that makes one susceptible to attack—these are, by far, the dominant themes. However, they do not tell the whole story, and in this essay I should like to probe one topic they leave obscure. I want to think about the role of contagion.

*

[2]Kanô, *Chûgoku igaku*, 67.

[3]Ibid., 67–8.

Where did contagion fit into this world of forces demonic and meteorological? At first blush, the answer might seem to be: not at all. It is possible to read a dozen modern accounts of Chinese medicine without encountering a single extended discussion of contagionism. Nor is this a historiographic quirk. Traditional Chinese doctors themselves put no emphasis on the subject.

Yet there is no doubt that people recognized the possibility of "catching" sickness. In his famous nosological compendium, the *Zhubing yuanhou zonglun* (610), Chao Yuanfang details numerous avenues of infection.

It is dangerous, for example, for a person suffering from open sores to mount a horse. For,

> the sweat, horsehairs, dirt, urine, and leather saddle blanket all can contain poisons. If the poisons enter the sore, they can cause inflamed swelling, aches and pains, fevers. If they enter the stomach, the person may die.[4]

It can happen, too, that one directly ingests poisons without knowing it, for under various circumstances even common foods go bad. Thus if a venomous snake spits venom on the grass, and the cow eats that grass, the cow will die and its meat will contain poison. Moreover,

> Cows which die of epidemic diseases (*yibing*) also contain poisons. If people eat their meat, they will suffer excruciating chest pains, extensive paralysis, vomiting, diarrhea, unbearable stomach cramps, and many will die.[5]

Much the same holds true for eating horses, birds, and other animals that have died from epidemics: all contain poisons that can make one very sick.[6]

Whether the poisons in the meat of the dead animals are the same poisons that killed the animal in the first place—whether in eating animals struck down by epidemic disease, one is eating the disease itself—these passages do not explicitly say, though their juxtaposition with the warning about snake venom is suggestive. In any case, dying from epidemic disease made the animals exceptionally noxious.

Then there are those diseases that pass directly from person to person. Wind, parasites, spirits, or sundry poisons may pour into young children or

[4] *ZBYHL*, *juan* 36, 143.

[5] Ibid., *juan* 26, 103.

[6] Ibid.

debilitated adults, and produce various *zhubing*, "influx diseases". Once inside, these pathogens roam around the body, causing swelling, fever, pain; or they lie dormant for long periods, causing death only after months or years. For us, the most notable point is this: when they kill one person, the deadly spirits or parasites then transfer themselves, and flow into someone nearby.[7] Even before a person dies, the noxious influx breath (*zhuqi*) can easily flow into those living with or looking after the patient, reproducing symptoms identical to those suffered by the patient.[8]

Nor are these the only communicable diseases. There are, Chao explains, actually two kinds of *shanghan*, or cold-damage disorders. One derives from the simple impact of the cold, and the illness does not affect others. But another arises when the seasons slip out of kilter, and the warm and the cold lose their regular order. The sickness of people succumbing to this circumstance, Chao says, is often contagious (*duo xiangran yi*).[9]

One Qing dynasty physician, Xiong Lipin, warned against approaching the bedding of those suffering from epidemic disease, because of the risk of infection from pollutants (*weiwu*). In a similar vein, he urged keeping one's distance from the corpse and coffin, and fleeing their noxious odors. Too, one should avoid eating the food at a sick person's home, or picking up a sick person's clothes. One modern historian has cited these suggestions as evidence of a new consciousness of contagion in Qing times.[10] But in fact these precautions are all traditional.

The people of Wu and Yue, Ge Hong reports in the *Baopuzi* (320), possess a method of special conjuration that fortifies the vital breath. So powerful is this method that, "He who knows it can pass safely through the worst epidemics, and even share a bed with a sick person without being infected."[11] The evident expectation in epidemics, then, was that those near the sick would normally also fall sick. The fact that one did not succumb, despite lying next to a patient, constituted strong evidence for the efficacy of the conjurations.

[7] Ibid., *juan* 47, 188. We glimpse here the close association of sickness and parasites. In Six Dynasty times, the term *wuyang*, literally, "to have no parasites," was a common phrase for good health.

[8] Ibid., *juan* 24, 96.

[9] *ZBYHZL*, *juan* 8, 38.

[10] Shi, "Shilun chuanranbing xuejia Wu Youke," 186 (see note 37 below).

[11] Cited in Joseph Needham, *China and the Origins of Immunology* (Hong Kong: University of Hong Kong, 1980), 11.

An anecdote in the official Jin dynasty history highlights contagionist expectations yet more forcefully. It tells of how near the end of the third century—shortly, therefore, after the time of Cao Zhi—a young man named Yu Gun lived through another serious epidemic. His two oldest brothers succumbed to the disease early on; a third brother fell gravely ill. As the epidemic gained momentum, Gun's parents and younger brothers evacuated the city, and urged Gun to leave with them. But Gun refused. He remained behind, alone, and nursed his sick brother day and night, foregoing sleep. When the brother finally died, Gun stroked his coffin with grief.

After a hundred days, the epidemic began to subside. The rest of the family returned, and marvelled to find Gun unharmed. "How strange!" they exclaimed. "This child has looked after what human beings cannot look after, and done what human beings cannot do." And "they began to suspect that epidemic disease is not contagious after all (*shi yi yili zhi bu xiangran ye*)".[12]

The compilers of this account do not commit themselves either to supporting or refuting this suspicion. But the story vividly illuminates the common understanding: the idea that epidemic disease (*yili*) is *not* contagious was an unexpected, startling possibility, contrary to conventional wisdom. Yu Gun's survival, despite prolonged proximity to his ailing brother, despite actually stroking his coffin—surely not an idle detail—provoked amazement. The sensible course was to flee.

The story may seem unremarkable to the modern reader, particularly if considered in isolation. There is, after all, no indication here of insights into specific pathogens, no attention to paths of transmission. There is only a vague, albeit powerful intuition that epidemic diseases spread easily, and that associating with the sick can be fatal. And this seems like a conclusion to which the actual experience of epidemics would almost inevitably lead.

Still, when considered in the context of the whole of Chinese medical culture, the story poses an intriguing puzzle. For it conjures up the image of a populace keenly conscious of the dangers of proximity to the sick; and this image contrasts sharply with what doctors wrote about epidemics. In the countless treatises that deal partly or exclusively with what we now think of contagious diseases, we encounter only faint traces of contagion consciousness. The overwhelming bulk of discourse on epidemics, we noted, focuses on the impact of the weather.

---

[12] *Jin shu*, "Yu Gun zhuan," (*SKQS*, vol. 256, 432)

Chao Yuanfang's compendium is no exception. He does refer, explicitly, to a contagious variety of *shanghan*. But this observation appears as the very last item in a discussion of *shanghan* that encompasses seventy-seven items in all. None of the other seventy-six items breathes a word about contagion. Moreover, the remarks I related above are about all he has to say about contagious *shanghan*. He advises taking medicine prophylactically, but he does not specify what that medicine should be; and he says nothing about how the epidemic is transmitted. He mentions contagion again with regard to *shiqibing* and *wenbing*, two other related ailments that cause epidemics. But in both these cases, too, the references appear only as brief remarks appended to long discussions of other matters.[13]

We glean some hints of how the nature and spread of epidemic disease was conceived, however, in the prophylactic advice offered by some later authors. In his *Introduction to medicine* (*Yixue rumen*, 1575), Li Ting suggests that a person entering a home afflicted by epidemic disease should either first ingest some sesame oil, or else twist some paper, steep the twisted ends in a mixture of sesame oil, orpiment (*xionghuang*), and cinnabar, and then use this paper to plug the nostrils and ears. These, he says, are the most effective means of averting polluting, poisonous influences (*weidu zhi qi*).[14]

Zhang Jiepin (1563–1640) traced warm-factor epidemics (*wenyi*) to fiery exhalations. When they accumulated in a home, the entire family would fall sick; accumulating in a village, they could afflict the entire prefecture; accumulating in a city, the entire metropolis; accumulating along the roadways, they might claim victims for a thousand *li* around. Much evidence suggests this, says Zhang, but the unfailing efficacy of purifying the area, and removing polluting substances offers clinching proof.[15]

For Zhang, too, the nose was crucial. Poisonous vapours entered through the nasal passages into the brain, and flowed from there through the conduits of breath and blood into the rest of the body. Sneezing or forcefully expelling breath through the nose, and then taking in deep breaths of pure air was one way of dispelling the poison. Another possibility was to burn aromatic incense. But the most proven method, according to Zhang, was to suck on biscuits made from Fujian aromatic tea.[16]

[13] *ZBYHL*, *juan* 9, 38; *juan* 10, 47.

[14] *Yixue rumen*, "Yili," (*YBQS*, 7137).

[15] *Jingyue quanshu*, "Wenyi zhifa," (*YBQS*, 7151).

[16] "Biyi fa", (*YBQS*, 7150–1). Similar measures can of course also be found in Europe. Thomas Willis recommends a series of substances that may be put in the nostrils, and others

As with much of the traditional literature in Europe, it is difficult, and often anachronistic to draw sharp distinctions between interpersonal contagion and shared miasmas. One became sick through *xiangran*, "mutual dyeing", or *chuanran*, "communicated dyeing": whether the noxious breath with which one became dyed was endemic to the area, or emanated from a particular individual was secondary. Sickness arrived along both routes. Noxious miasmas (*zhangqi*) emanated from the ground, or sometimes from the bodies of dead rats. But one had to take precautions too, against vapours issuing from the already sick.

One Ming-period doctor advanced the strange, but striking notion that noxious breath emanates, in the case of men, from the mouth, and in the case of women, from the genitals. The reasoning behind this distinction is unclear, but his conclusion leaves no doubt that he imagined the poisonous effluvia as something quite concrete, issuing from particular places in a particular direction:

> When encountering [patients], therefore, one must always be conscious of whether one is looking at them face to face, or facing away from them. Alternatively, if one coats the nasal passages with orpiment, then one can move around freely.... It is essential that physicians entering the home of the sick bear these things in mind.[17]

People knew, then, that those sick with certain ailments could pass their sickness onto others. And they took precuations. They ingested medicines. They sucked on special biscuits. They blocked the nasal passages, or coated them with antitoxins. They evacuated to the countryside, far away from the ailing. If we look hard enough, we can find considerably more and stronger evidence of contagion-consciousness than the secondary literature on Chinese medicine has generally lead us to expect.

---

that one can chew as protection in passing through plague-infested regions (*A plain and easie method for preserving [by God's blessing] those that are well from inflection of the plague or any other contagious distemper* [London, 1691], 20–2). The persisting association of odours and sickness in the eighteenth and nineteenth centuries is vividly evoked in Alain Corbin's, *The Foul and the Fragrant* (Harvard University Press, 1986).

Not all prevention focused on respiration. According to Sun Simiao's *Qianjin yaofang* (seventh century), officials going to the regions of Wu and Shu made sure always to keep several unhealed moxibustion sores on their bodies. This, they believed, protected them from the epidemics endemic to these regions.

[17] Cited in *Jingyue quanshu*, *juan* 13, "Biyi fa," (*SKQS*, vol. 777, 265).

The point that must be stressed, however, is that we have to ferret out this evidence. It appears scattered in incidental observations, matter-of-fact remarks about the different kinds of disease, and the precautions that some require. Although the story of Yu Gun intimates a vivid consciousness of contagion among the general population, this consciousness never appears at the forefront of doctors' concerns, as a major preoccupation. Traditional Chinese medical literature offers no extended systematic attempts to analyse the nature and means of disease transmission. The central fact about contagionism in traditional Chinese medical thought is not its absence, but its relative obscurity.

How should we understand this obscurity? In his classic article on the contagionist-anticontagionist debate in nineteenth-century Europe, Erwin Ackerknecht pointed out how the debate was never just an argument about aetiology—how, that is, accepting the reality of contagion implied preventive measures with dramatic social and economic consequences. Many people had much to lose if contagionism triumphed and quarantine were imposed.[18] During the Wellcome conference it was hypothesized, in a similar vein, that one disincentive against a more developed discourse of contagion in certain traditional cultures may have been that the isolation of the sick was either unfeasible or unpalatable, or both.

But in the case of traditional China, there is little evidence to encourage such an interpretation. No doctor ever explicitly denied the possibility of contagion, and many freely conceded it a role in certain diseases. When entering an epidemic-stricken home, doctors routinely took precautions. The phenomenon of contagion was widely recognized; only it remained, somehow, a distant, peripheral concern. To repeat: the puzzle that we confront concerns neither the denial of contagion nor a failure to notice it. The question, rather, is why so little was made of it.

*

The basic answer, I believe, is simple. It is that contagion never loomed large in the traditional analysis of epidemics because other factors seemed more critical. Contagionism was not so much played down as overshadowed. Chinese physicians were preoccupied with other concerns. Invariably, and at length,

---

[18] Erwin Ackerknecht, "Anticontagionism between 1821 and 1867," *Bulletin of the History of Medicine* 22 (1948): 562–93.

their treatises lingered on the ravages of wind and cold, heat, humidity, dryness. It was especially on the claims of weather that the fate of contagionism in China turned.

Modern accounts of Chinese medicine often convey the impression that the primary concern of Chinese physicians was balance—balance in the foods that a person ate, in the feelings that a person felt, in the activities that filled a life; that health, in the Chinese view, hinged on harmony among the forces in the body and in the surrounding cosmos; that sickness was essentially imbalance. Though these accounts regularly mention cold and heat and the like as factors that upset the body's balance, they usually fail to convey both the intensity of the traditional preoccupation with weather, and the range of afflictions for which it was blamed.

Yet the "Medicine" volumes of the encyclopedic *Gujin tushu jicheng* opens its exposition of the causes of disease with no less than eight *juan* (more than 700 pages of the original edition) just to disorders caused by wind. And this mirrors the mainstream. Treatise after Chinese treatise exhaustively details the maladies, astonishingly numerous and diverse, wrought by the weather—and these include, of course, virtually all epidemic diseases. Balance was a concern, to be sure. One's emotions lose their keel, one eats too much, one exhausts oneself in sexual dissipation—all Chinese doctors agreed that these predisposed toward sickness. But the space actually devoted to the effects of poor regimen and the swings and swerves of feeling is pitifully thin when compared to the enormous bulk of discourse lavished on wind and cold, heat, humidity, and dryness—their impact, diagnosis, and treatment.

Let me be clear. I am not suggesting that external factors mattered more than internal predispositions. Such a formulation is plainly false: the principle that pathogens like wind and cold hurt only the already debilitated—that a person's inner vigor ultimately determines the harm, or harmlessness, of outer forces—remained an unwavering conviction of all traditional physicians.[19]

---

[19] *Suwen* 1 and *Lingshu* 66 present canonical expressions of this notion. Zhang Jiepin, for his part, observed:

> Now *wenbing* epidemics are due to the harmful emanations of heaven and earth. But if a person's vital breath is firm inside, then the harmful influences cannot invade and infect. Thus, the key to averting them lies in moderating one's desires and exertions. (*Jingyue quanshu, juan* 13 "Biyi fa" [*SKQS*, vol. 777, 264]).

I am pointing out, however, that weather riveted the attention of Chinese physicians to an extent, and in a way, that is hard for us now to understand, and that we often fail fully to appreciate. Yet to the extent that we neglect this rivetting of attention we risk both misjudging the overall character of Chinese medicine, and misreading in particular the traditional stance toward contagion.

Two points cannot be stressed enough. The first is that the issue of weather, and especially of weather and epidemics, was inseparable from the problem of seasonality, and the problem of seasonality was in essence the problem of cosmic order. Spring should be warm, summer hot, autumn cool, winter cold: on this rhythm rested the growth and flourishing of the harvest, the prosperity of the empire, the health of the people. Epidemics sprang not so much from imbalance as irregularity, not from excess heat or cold, but heat or cold *at the wrong time*. If summer got too hot, or winter too cold, people might well fall prey to sundry illnesses, but they rarely died suddenly, and in masses. Sweeping, virulent, fatal sicknesses broke out when seasonal expectations were thwarted, when winter was balmy, say, or summer brisk and chilly. Cao Zhi, recall, attributed the epidemics of his age not to cold or heat per se, but to the "confusion of the *yin* and the *yang*"—coolness and warmth arriving out of turn. From the Han dynasty through the Qing, this belief remained the mainstay of the *shanghan* view of epidemics: the deadliest ailments sprang from seasons out of kilter.

The menace of weather, therefore, was not just or even primarily a matter of the violence of wind or rain, sun or freezing cold, by themselves, as brute forces. It was not just that in an age before electricity, modern heating, and air-conditioning, climate intruded more inescapably into people's daily lives—though it undoubtedly did. The really crucial issue was *when* winds blew hot or cold, *when* it rained or did not. The heart of the matter was the regularity or irregularity of seasonal succession.[20]

Understood in this way, the centrality of meterology in Chinese medicine—and along with it, the peripheral obscurity of contagionism—seem almost inevitable. They mirrored the traditional faith in a coherent, intimate, interrelated universe, a faith which, articulated through the corres-pondances of *yin* and *yang* and the five phases, dominated not just think-

[20] I have discussed the evolution of the connections between time, sickness, and wind in, "The imagination of winds, and the development of the Chinese conception of the body," in Angela Zito and Tani Barlow eds., *Body, Subject, and Power in China* (Chicago: University of Chicago Press, 1994), 23–41.

ing about the relationship of human beings to sickness, but their relationships to the cosmos, to each other, and to their deepest moral selves. Doctors and laymen alike, we've noted, had no doubt that some deadly diseases could be caught from the sick, and they took measures to fend off contamination. But in the end, this awareness of contagion amounted to scarcely more than occasional observations about a few diseases. Unlike the aetiology of untimely weather, they did not form part—and thus lacked the reverberating resonance—of a comprehensive worldview.

We readily recognize in *shanghan* analysis what Charles Rosenberg has called the configuration—as opposed to the contamination—explanation of epidemics.[21] This type of explanation, which traces sudden, widespread sicknesses to disruptions in the holistic ecology of human beings and the world, was of course hardly unique to China. It held sway in many cultures, including the traditional West. That certain climatic conditions and illnesses are proper to each season; that the illness accompanying regular seasons are themselves regular and easy to manage; that irregular weather spawns irregular illnesses that are hard to cure—such ideas appear also and already in Hippocrates.[22] Even in the nineteenth century, many in Europe and America still spoke of epidemic constitutions.

We must take care, however, not to assimilate too quickly. To elucidate the precise nuances of the history of contagionism in China, we must attend to divergences as well as parallels. This brings me to my second point: although both traditional European and Chinese doctors regularly traced sickness to weather, they conceived weather's impact in quite separate ways.

Weather in Galenic analysis was mainly a *causa procatarctica*, an initial cause.[23] Wind and cold harmed the body indirectly, by altering the tension or laxity of the fibres, by damaging the flow and equilibrium of the humours, by jolting the body's delicate balance. In China, by contrast, weather intruded straight into the body. Instead of just instigating harmful inner change, as external stimuli, wind and cold were, in a sense, the disease itself.

---

[21] Charles Rosenberg, "Explaining epidemics," in his *Explaining Epidemics and Other Studies in the History of Medicine* (Cambridge: Cambridge University Press, 1992), 293–304.

[22] See Georghe Bratescu, "Aspects d'étiologie dans les Épidémies hippocratiques," in Gerhard Baader and Rolf Winau eds., *Die hippokratischen Epidemien. Theorie-Praxis-Tradition. Verhandlungen des Ve Colloque International Hippocratique.* (Stuttgart: Franz Steiner Verlag, 1989), 222–36.

[23] Vivian Nutton, "The seeds of disease: an explanation of contagion and infection from the Greeks to the Renaissance," *Medical History* 27 (1983), 4.

In her critique of the metaphors of attack and infiltration so prominent in modern medicine, Susan Sontag suggests that, "The military metaphor in medicine came into wide use in the 1880s, with the identification of bacteria as agents of disease."[24] She speaks, presumably, with only the West in mind. Some two thousand years earlier, the *Huangdi neijing* boiled down the bare essentials of pathology to *xu* and *shi*, depletion and fullness. These are often glossed, today, as reflecting the equation of sickness and imbalance. But the logic that actually inspired and sustained them was not that of exceeding or falling short of some ideal mean, but rather, the paradigm of war. *Shi* was the excess of a body occupied by foreign intruders, *xu* was the emptiness that made intrusion possible. The former was the surfeit of *exogenous* pathogens, the latter was the lack of *endogenous* vitality.[25] *Xu* and *shi* were thus not polarized alternatives, but rather stages in a causal sequence: depletion within the body invited invasion from without.[26]

Patients in traditional China are "wounded" (*shang*) by cold, "hit" (*zhong*) by wind; physicians deploy acupuncture and medicines to "attack" (*gong*) the disease; sickness is siege. The distant origins of this way of imagining sickness may well lie in the archaic medicine of spirit possession and expulsion. The two ways of explaining epidemics that I distinguished at the outset may thus have common roots. In any case, martial analogies continued to flourish long after classical writings shifted blame from demons to climate. The Ming doctor Tao Hua (1369–1450), for example, explained,

> The way in which one's vital breath is harmed by the approach of polluted breath is just like this: when the walls and barriers [of a fortress] are not solid, bandits dare to enter. If one's vitality is strong, pathogenic influences have difficulty invading.[27]

Once upon a time, recounts Wu Youxing (1580s–1660s), three people were assaulted by the same mist. "The one with the empty stomach died, the one who had drunk wine became ill, the one who had eaten his fill did

---

[24]Susan Sontag, *Illness as Metaphor* (New York: Vintage Books, 1979), 65.

[25]*Suwen* Chapter 28, 86; Chapter 53, 145. The pages refer to Ren Yingqiu's indexed edition, *Huangdi neijing zhangju suoyin* (Taipei: Qiye shuju, 1987).

[26]For a more detailed discussion of the themes of depletion and fullness—and how they relate to a comparison of classical Chinese and Greek medicine—see my "Interpreting the history of bloodletting," *Journal of the History of Medicine and Allied Sciences* 50 (1995): 11–46.

[27]Tao Hua, *Quansheng ji*, "Shiqi," (*YBQS*, 7136).

not even become sick." The principle was simple: when one is full of vital energy, pathogens cannot enter; only when that energy is depleted and deficient do noxious influences rush in.[28]

Yet it is especially in the vision of what happens after the walls are breached that the full force of the image becomes clear. For wind and cold did not just intrude. They wandered. And as they wandered, lodging now in one organ now in another, different functions became impaired, different parts ached. The *Shanghan lun* and its commentaries explore the subtle patterns governing these movements and their consequences. But the core intuition, from antiquity, was that of progressive penetration.

First breaching the skin and pores, the sickening influences gradually burrowed deeper—into the conduits, the sinews, the flesh, into the hollow organs, into the solid organs, into the very marrow of the bones.[29]

---

[28] *WYLP*, 11.

[29] This intuition appears already in the most famous story of Chinese medical legend, Bian Que's diagnosis of Duke Huan. The version in the 105th chapter of Sima Qian's *Historical records* (composed between 104–91 BCE) runs as follows:

> Bian Que passed through the country of Qi. The Duke of Qi invited him to be his guest. Received by the Duke, Bian Que warned him, "My Lord has an ailment which lies in the pores. If it is not treated, it will penetrate deeper." Duke Huan replied, "I am not sick." Bian Que left. Duke Huan remarked to his attendants, "Physicians are greedy. They want to take credit for curing people who are not even sick."
>
> Five days later, Bian Que was received again. He warned the Duke, "My Lord has an ailment which lies in the blood vessels. If it is not treated, I fear it will penetrate deeper." The Duke replied, "I am not sick." Bian Que left. The Duke was displeased.
>
> Five days later, Bian Que was received again. He urged the Duke, "My Lord has an ailment which lies in the stomach and intestines. If it is not treated, it will penetrate deeper." Duke Huan did not respond. Bian Que left. Duke Huan was displeased.
>
> Five days later, Bian Que was received again. Gazing at Duke Huan from a distance, he retreated and rushed rapidly away. The Duke sent a man to ask Bian Que about the reasons for his behaviour. Bian Que explained, "When the disease lies in the pores, it can be treated by poultices. When it lies in the blood vessels, it can be treated with needles. When it lies in the stomach and intestines, it can be treated with medicines. But when the disease lies in the bone marrow, not even the God of Life can do anything about it. The Duke's disease now lies in the bone marrow, and it is for this that I have no more advice."

When they still hovered near the pores and vessels they might be expelled by poultices, sudorifics, or acupuncture; but if that opportunity was lost, and the disease sank in, these treatments might only sap the patient's own vitality. To attack the disease at that stage, emetics might be required; or, if the invaders penetrated yet further, diuretics and purgatives might be called for. The paradigm of invasion thus had direct, practical implications. It framed diagnosis. It guided therapy. Fundamental to judging any disease was determining whether it was lodged near the surface (*biao*), or deep inside (*li*), or midway inbetween (*banbiao banli*).[30]

There is a gap, then, between our current common perceptions of Chinese etiological thought, and the historical reality. The former revolve, monotonously, on holistic themes—harmony and disharmony, balance and imbalance.[31] But historically, Chinese doctors saw sickness at least as often in terms of vulnerability and intrusion. Cold and wind attacked, swept in, migrated, bore deeper toward a person's vital core, as if they were discrete entities, grim invaders, disease itself. In this, they resembled more the bacteria of the

[30]One further example. No diagnostic technique claimed more attention, traditionally, than the palpation of the pulse. But Chinese pulse analysis was framed by a basic distinction alien to Galenic sphygmology—the distinction between the "floating" (*fu*) and the "sunken" (*chen*). This distinction corresponded to the difference between diseases or vital energies concentrated near the surface (*biao*), and those lodged deep in the interior (*li*). The fifth "difficulty" (*nan*) of the *Nanjing* suggests yet more refined distinctions: the pulse felt superficially, with minimal pressure (literally, with the weight of three beans) reveals the state of the skin and pores and the organ which governs them, namely, the lungs; slightly deeper (felt with the pressure of six beans), the pulse expresses the state of the blood-vessels and their governing organ, the heart; a third level corresponds to the flesh and spleen, a fourth level to the tendons and liver, and the deepest level, felt with the pressure of fifteen beans, reveals the condition of the bones, and their principal organ, the kidneys.

[31]The history of recent representations of traditional Chinese medicine is notable for the exoticist bias of these representations—the tendency to highlight precisely those elements of traditional Chinese medicine that ostensibly make it alien to contemporary Western notions, to polarize Western and Chinese approaches, and to portray the latter as the opposite, or at least the complement, of the former. We see it expressed most commonly in the oppositions of Chinese organicism to Western mechanism, Chinese stress on holistic balance to Western warfare against pathogens. Dissatisfaction with contemporary Western biomedicine is one obvious factor behind this trend; another is a longer history of Orientalism in which dismissals of a hopelessly backward Asia, have alternated with the romantic quest to recover in Asia the really deep truths somehow lost sight of in the West. Asian self-portrayals, for their part, have also often stressed difference as one strategy of self-affirmation.

A subtler factor that deserves closer scrutiny is how modern Western visions of the exotic otherness of traditional Chinese medicine have been filtered through the assumptions of traditional Western medicine. The stress on physiological balance may be a case in point.

modern imagination than climate in Galenic humoralism. Weather and its influence can be and was conceived in very different ways. Meteorological medicine is not simple, single, everywhere the same.

A moment ago, I cited Tao Hua's analysis of how the "polluted breaths" (*weiqi*) that caused epidemics infiltrated the body, like bandits rushing in through crumbling walls. A long Western tradition disposes us, upon hearing the term "pollution", immediately to imagine dirt and impurities, miasmas and foul smells.[32] And certainly such associations were not absent in China—recall, for instance, Zhang Jiepin's remarks on the prophylactic efficacy of incense and aromatic biscuits. Yet, is also certain that the emphases of Chinese and European doctors were not the same.

From Galen's "pestilential seeds" (*loimou spermata*), through the persisting fears about corrupt, vitiated air, to the nineteenth-century research that led to the theory of "germs", European reflection upon epidemics returned insistently to images of putrefaction, fermentation, corruption. The leitmotiv of Chinese aetiology, by contrast, was intrusion, and pollution often referred as much to temporal irregularity as to material corruption. The polluting assailant in Tao Hua's portrait of siege was not "matter out of place," to echo Mary Douglas' famous formula, but rather "time out of order," not putrid exhalations, but unseasonal influences (*shiqi*)–cold in summer, heat in winter.[33] The polluted breath that swept into and attacked the body's innate vitality was chaotic time, conceived as a real, noxious, contagious stream.

Li Ting, we may remember, urged doctors entering epidemic-afflicted households to stuff paper steeped in sesame oil and orpiment into the ears and nose. But in the sentence immediately preceding this prescription, he quotes the *Neijing*: "In dealing with epidemic breaths, do not rely on diagnostic inspection, but seek the answer rather in the circulation of breaths (*yunqi*)."[34] The circulation of breaths was the theory that rooted human health in the dialectic of the *yin* and the *yang*, the cycle of the five phases, the alternation of six seasonal influences. It delineated how different sicknesses sprang from disordered time. His prophylactic advice makes clear, however, that disordered

---

[32] On the early religious implications, see Robert Parker, *Miasma. Pollution and Purification in Early Greek Religion* (Oxford: Clarendon Press, 1983).

[33] The course of disease caused by this *shiqi*, Tao tells us, is similar to that caused by *shanghan*. But *shanghan* is caused by harm from cold; in *shiqi* (disease) one is afflicted by epidemic breath (*yili zhi qi*). It cannot be treated in the same way. (Tao Hua, *Quansheng ji*, "Shiqi," [*YBQS*, 7136]).

[34] Li Ting, *Yixue rumen*, "Yili," (*YBQS*, 7137).

time for Li Ting was not just an analytical abstraction. It was a palpable presence, a disease that entered through the body's orifices, an influence that could be blocked by plugging the ears and nostrils.

I alluded above to Charles Rosenberg's distinction between the configuration and contamination explanations of epidemics. Rosenberg himself concedes the porousness of the divide, and Chinese medicine provides a striking illustration. Unseasonal weather constituted, clearly, a disruption in the cosmic order; yet at the same time it could also pollute, and pass on to others. For Chao Yuanfang, for Li Ting, for Zhang Jiepin, unseasonal cold differed from cold in winter not only by its greater virulence, but by its communicability. Meterological pathology in China did not merely overshadow contagionism. It pinpointed the most potent contagious influences.

*

Like Zhang Ji some fourteen hundred years earlier, Wu Youxing lived in a time of frequent epidemics.[35] His contemporaries still treated these as cold-damage disorders, and churned out commentary after commentary on the *Shanghan lun*. Wu felt sure that they were wrong.

Out of every hundred patients diagnosed as victims of *shanghan*, he came to believe, only a tiny fraction—one or two perhaps—were really afflicted by cold-damage. The overwhelming majority suffered from causes overlooked by doctors in the past. Their illnesses came not from cold or wind or heat or humidity, nor even from faulty regimen or draining emotions—though these latter made one vulnerable. The true origins of sickness lay, rather, in diverse, heterogeneous *qi*, *zaqi*—specific pathogens inducing specific kinds of disease.[36] Prior to the turn toward Western medicine in late Qing times, no one challenged the received wisdom more radically.

In an early article on Wu Youxing as a "theorist of contagious diseases" (*chuanranbing xuejia*), the Chinese scholar Shi Changlong touted Wu's theory of *zaqi* as the beginnings of a move toward modernity, a prescient intuition of germ theory, and he marveled at how the Ming dynasty doctor anticipated Pasteur by some two hundred years.[37] We tend, today, to be wary of such assimilations. We know how easily present assumptions distort past beliefs, and

[35] Helen Dunstan, "The late Ming epidemics: a preliminary survey," *Ch'ing-shih wen-t'i* 3.3 (Nov. 1975): 1–59.

[36] *WYLP*, 332–9.

[37] Shi Changyong, "Shilun chuanranbing xuejia Wu Youke ji qi liqi xueshuo," *Yixueshi yu baojian zuzhi* 1957 no. 3: 180–6. I should like to thank Dr. Carol Benedict of Williams College

we cannot but suspect that assimilating across cultures will double the distortion. Vivian Nutton has shown how the interpretation of Fracastoro as a revolutionary forerunner of germ theory misreads the development of European discourse on disease.[38] Speaking of Wu Youxing as a Chinese Fracastoro consequently seems all the more problematic.[39]

In fact what makes Wu Youxing so interesting for our study is precisely the irrelevance of the issue of contagion to his rebellion against orthodoxy. Yes, *zaqi* could pass from person to person.[40] But so could, traditionally, unseasonal weather. Yes, *zaqi* entered the body through the nose and mouth, instead of filtering through the skin like wind and cold. But older contemporaries like Li Ting and Zhang Jiepin already supposed epidemic diseases to spread through inspired air. In the history of Western aetiology, the move from tradition toward modernity is closely associated with the shift from a holistic conception of sickness as physiological imbalance, focused on the individual, to an ontological conception of disease as the intrusion of specific, alien pathogens.[41] But in the tradition against which Wu rebelled, untimely heat and cold, wind, humidity, dryness already figured as transgressors from the outside, penetrating, contagious. Anyone contemplating a comparative history of contagion must bear this lesson in mind: weather and its impact can be conceived in many ways. Meteorological medicine is neither simple, nor everywhere the same.

Wu's break with meteorological orthodoxy challenged, above all, the hegemony of cosmic time. Traditionally, the workings of the body, the workings of the state, and workings of the earth and heavens could all be reduced to the rhythms of the *yin* and the *yang*, the five phases, seasonal change. In Wu Youxing's vision, on the other hand, things possessed their own, independent possibilities of action, properties irreducible to complementary pairs or groups of five, potencies that exerted their influence regardless of whether it was spring or summer, autumn or winter. Some diseases struck cows but not

for alerting me to, and providing me with copies of this article and the Chinese articles cited in note 44. Further, Dr. Benedict's own manuscripts on the history of plague in China have helped me to crystallize my thinking about weather and contagion.

[38] Nutton, "The seeds of disease," 1–34.

[39] Shi, "Shilun," 186.

[40] *WYLP*, 11.

[41] Owsei Temkin, "The scientific approach to disease: specific entity and individual sickness," in A. C. Crombie, *Scientific Change* (London: Heinemann, 1963): 629–47; Christopher Hamlin, "Predisposing causes and public health in early nineteenth-century medical thought," *Social History of Medicine* 5 (1992): 43–70.

sheep. Some afflicted humans but not animals. Slugs dissolved the toxin of the poisonous centipede. Cat's meat healed ulcerating rat bites. For each kind of *qi* that made one sick, there was another kind of *qi* to counteract it.[42] In place of a universe ruled by a few overarching principles, Wu pictured a far more complex world of specific sympathies and antipathies. *Zaqi* belonged to no direction or season. They could strike anywhere, at any time.[43]

The sources and motivations of Wu's theory, and the impact of his thought on the subsequent development of Chinese medicine, lie outside the scope of this essay.[44] We know, in any case, that he did not dramatically alter the mainstream: the emphasis on the connection between disease and seasonality continued to dominate thinking about epidemics for centuries afterward. And this is not surprising. Meteorological aetiology supported and was supported by a vision of a unified, coherent cosmos. One could not challenge the paradigm of seasonal climates without ultimately calling into question the received understanding of society, of the state, of the workings of heaven and earth. The implications of doubt were huge.

The introduction to one modern edition of the *Wenyilun* presents the theory of *zaqi* as a revolutionary attack on the conservative feudal order.[45] Whereas the old pathology of cosmic irregularity made epidemics inevitable, suggest the editors, and left the people passive and powerless against the will of Heaven, Wu posited discrete, material enemies that might be combated, actively, by specific material remedies. The edition appeared in 1977, and the ideological imprint of the Cultural Revolution (1966–76) is obvious. Still, given the undeniable intertwining of conceptions of bodily, political, and cosmic disorder this suggestion may merit more detailed analysis.

Another factor contributing, perhaps, to the stability of the meteorological paradigm—though this hypothesis too needs more careful study—may have been the ties between medical doctrine and professional identity. In-

---

[42] *WYLP*, 210.

[43] *WYLP*, 196.

[44] Gao Hesheng, "Cong Wu Youke, Ye Tianshi, Wu Jutong sanjia xhueshuo kan wenbingxue de fazhan," *Zhejiang zhongyi yao* July 1979: 225–8 reviews Wu's place in the development of the theory of *wenbing*, or "warm-factor" diseases. On the development of *wenbing* more generally, see Deng Tietao, "Wenbing xueshuo de fasheng yu chengzhang," *Zhongyi zazhi* 1955, no. 5: 6–10; Shi Yiren, "Wenbing fazhan jianshi," *Zhonghua yishi zazhi* 1955, no. 4: 259–62. All these will likely be superseded by the work of Marta Hansen, *Inventing a Tradition in Chinese Medicine: from Universal Canon to Medical Knowledge in South China, Seventeenth to the Nineteenth Century*, Ph.D. thesis, University of Pennsylvania (1997).

[45] *WYLP*, 4.

terpreting diseases as reflections of sweeping, universal transformations made physicians experts in a science from which they presumably could claim much more prestige (and derive more self-esteem) than from knowledge of scattered, mundane, miscellaneous *qi*. This may, more generally, be a significant part of the answer to the enigmatic obscurity of contagion in traditional China—the puzzling disparity between the apparently widespread popular awareness of contagion, and the absence of a sustained discourse on contagion in the medical literature. The silence may owe not a little, that is, to the incentives for physicians, particularly physicians with the education, status, and ambition to compose and publish enduring treatises, to spotlight those grand principles defining medicine as a cosmic science.

My main argument, in any case, is that we need to revise our current conceptions of this science. We need, for one, to rethink it as a science ruled as much by martial images of siege and invasion as by the holistic ideals of balance and harmony. We need, for another, to recognize more fully the extraordinary menace associated with the weather. And not least, we need to appreciate seasonality in Chinese medicine as a palpable influence, intrusive, and sometimes contagious.

Key to characters

banbiao banli 半表半裏
Baopuzi 抱朴子
biao 表
Cao Zhi 曹植
Chao Yuanfang 巢元方
chen 沈
Chen Yan 陳言
chuanran 傳染
chuanranbing xuejia 傳染病學家
duo xiangran yi 多相染易
fu 浮
Ge Hong 葛洪
gong 攻
Gujin tushu jicheng 古今圖書集成
Huangdi neijing 黃帝內經
li 裏
Li Ting 李梴
ligui 癘鬼
nan 難
Nanjing 難經
shang 傷
shanghan 傷寒
Shanghan lun 傷寒論
shi 實
shi yi yili zhi bu xiangran ye 始疑疫癘之不相染也
Shiming 釋名
Shiqi 時氣
shiqibing 時氣病
Sun Simiao 孫思邈
Tao Hua 陶華

weidu zhi qi 穢毒之氣
weiqi 穢氣
weiwu 穢物
wenbing 瘟病
wenyi 瘟疫
Wu Youxing 吳有性
wuyang 無恙
xiangran 相染
Xiong Lipin 熊立品
xionghuang 雄黃
xu 虛
yi (corvée) 役
yi (epidemics) 疫
yibing 疫病
yili 疫癘
Yitong 醫統
Yixue rumen 醫學入門
Yu Gun 庾袞
yunqi 運氣
zaqi 雜氣
Zhang Ji 張機
Zhang Jiepin 張介賓
zhangqi 瘴氣
Zheng Xuan 鄭玄
zhong 中
zhubing 注病
zhuqi 注氣

2

Dispersing the Foetal Toxin of the Body: Conceptions of Smallpox Aetiology in Pre-modern China

Chia-Feng Chang

The received biomedical conception of "contagion" refers to the spread of disease caused by someone coming into contact with, or close proximity to another person who is already affected by the disease. In the pre-modern world, however, different cultures held diverse views of the origin of disease. These views demonstrate various aspects of medical systems, and how people thought about disease.

In this paper I should like to introduce theories of the causes of smallpox which developed through several centuries in pre-modern China. I will then put these theories into a wider context of traditional Chinese medicine, discussing them and some related theoretical problems. In so doing, we can see different concepts of a contagious disease in traditional Chinese medicine.

Although the date of the first emergence of smallpox in China remains in debate,[1] the earliest surviving report of a large-scale outbreak of smallpox

---

I am grateful for Dr. Christopher Cullen's valuable comments on my draft and also for the criticism of Professor Nathan Sivin, Dr. Marta Hanson, Dr. Joanna Grant, John P. C. Moffett, and Professor Tim Barrett.

[1]The *Zhou hou bei ji fang*, which was written by Ge Hong (281–341), is the earliest surviving medical text which refers to the first large-scale smallpox outbreak in pre-modern China. However, the episode it mentions is not clearly dated. According to this account, soldiers fought a foreign enemy, and some of them contracted smallpox in the "*jian wu*" period. But there are several reign periods named "*jian wu*" before or during the author's life time, so the exact chronology of the "*jian wu*" period remains a matter of debate.

See Fan Xingzhun, *Zhong guo yu fang yi xue shi* (Beijing: Ren Min Wei Sheng Chu Ban She, 1953), 106–10; Li Jingwei, "Ji Zai Tian Hua Zui Zao Wen Xian De Bian Zheng," *Guang dong yi xue* (1964): 35–8.

dates from the fourth century AD.[2] The writer of this medical account noted that if the patients were not treated immediately, they would soon die. He also noticed that the pock-marks usually remained for one year, and assumed that it was caused by a noxious and poisonous form of *qi* (*e'du zhi qi*). This may be the earliest stage in the history of Chinese encounters with this dreadful disease.

In 610, when Chao Yuanfang complied a medical text, the *Zhu bing yuan hou lun* ("Compilation on the Origins of Disorders"), which was concerned with the origins and symptoms of disorders, he classified smallpox under four of his various categories of disease, cold-damage disorders (*shang han*), seasonal vapour (*shi qi*), hot disorders (*re bing*), and epidemic (*yi li bing*). He thought that smallpox was caused by over-accumulated heat toxin (*re du*), which originated from being hurt by cold in winter, or by unseasonable *qi*, and implied that smallpox could break out at any time.[3] Later in the Tang Dynasty (618–907), smallpox was mainly treated as cold-damage disorder or an epidemic disease.[4] During the Sui and Tang periods (589–907), physicians categorized smallpox by its various symptoms (*hou*), and it could thus be found in the different divisions of aetiology in medical texts.

From the Five Dynasties and the Song and Yuan period (907–1368) onwards, smallpox was gradually regarded as a paediatric disease. In the course of periodic smallpox outbreaks, a large proportion of the population was progressively affected, and thereby immunized against it. Year after year, the average age of new patients decreased, and children became the main sufferers. Many physicians, such as Pang Anshi (1043–1110?) and Liu Fang (?–1150), reported that smallpox was often rampant, with devastating consequences,[5] and as Zhang Gao, a physician, noted in the twelfth century, children rarely

[2] Ge Hong (281–341), *Zhou hou bei ji fang*, reprint of Zheng tong dao zang edition (Shanghai: Shang Wu Yin Shu Guan, 1955), *juan* 2, 235–36. The *Zhou hou bei ji fang* also reported that smallpox was spreading from the west to the east in the fourth year of the "*yong hui*" regnal period. However, there was no reign entitled "*yong hui*" prior to or during Ge Hong's and Tao Hingjing's lifetime. Therefore, the exact date of the fourth year of this period is also in doubt. For further details, see *ibid.*

[3] Chao Yuanfang, ed., *Zhu bing yuan hou lun*, re-edited by Ding Guangdi, (Beijing: Ren Min Wei Sheng Chu Ban She, 1992), *juan* 7, 236–37; *juan* 9, 295; *juan* 9, 312; *juan* 10, 336.

[4] Sun Simiao, *Qian jin bei ji yao fang* (652) (Taipei: Taiwan Shang Wu Yin Shu Guan, 1986), *juan* 32, 5–7; Wang Tao, *Wai tai mi yao fang* (752) (Taipei: Taiwan Shang Wu Yin Shu Guan, 1986), *juan* 3, 38.

[5] Pang Anshi, *Shang han zong bing lun* (Taipei: Taiwan Shang Wu Yin Shu Guan, 1986), *juan* 4, 11–12; Liu Fang, *You you xin shu* (1150) (Beijing: Ren Ming Wei Sheng Chu Ban She, 1987), *juan* 18, 660–661.

escaped.[6] As a result of this, a number of medical theories about the origins of smallpox in children and its treatment were developed. This new and crucial development on smallpox aetiology were later followed by physicians in the Ming and Qing periods (1368–1911).

After the Five Dynasties and Song period, the prevalent theory concerning smallpox aetiology was based on the concept of "foetal toxin" (*tai du*), heat toxin given to the infant by its mother, or father, or by both. Many physicians considered that since the infant relied on its mother to gain nutrition during pregnancy, it may have absorbed contaminated blood or liquid from its mother's visceral systems (*zang fu*). The contaminated matter which contained the heat toxin would be stored in the so-called *ming men* (gate of life) of the foetus as *tai du*.[7] *Ming men* was regarded as the fountain of life, and as the organ which stored the elements essential for conceiving children.[8] The *tai du* remained quiescent in the *ming men*; only becoming active when triggered by certain external factors, and then the patient developed smallpox.

Physicians believed that contaminated matter left in the mouth of the newborn infant was visible as blood and mucus. If the mother wiped them away immediately, the *tai du* would not enter into the infant's body.[9] After removing the contaminated matter, the infant had also to be given medicine to make sure that no *tai du* had been stored in its body.[10] This method was frequently mentioned in many medical texts, and was regarded as an important procedure in caring for newborn infants.[11] It was supposed to protect newborn

---

[6] Zhong Gao, *Yi shuo* (1189) (Taipei: Taiwan Shang Wu Yin Shu Guan, 1986), *juan* 10, 9.

[7] Qian Yi, *Xiao-er yao zheng zhi jue* (1093) (Beijing: Ren Ming Wei Sheng Chu Ban She, 1955), *juan* 1, 15. There are various suggestions about the location of *ming men*; it might be the right or left kidney, a body between the kidneys, or an immaterial locus of vital *qi*. For details, see Chia-Feng Chang, "Sheng Hua Zhi Yuan Yu Li Ming Zhi Men- Jin Yuan Ming Yi Xue Zhong De Ming Men Shi Tan", unpublished paper presented in the 'Medicine and Chinese Society' symposium at the Academia Sinica, Taipei, 1997.

[8] Li Gao (1180–1251), *Lan shi mi cang*, (Shanghai: Shanghai Gu Ji Chu Ban She, 1987), *juan* 2, 69.

[9] Ibid., 69–70.

[10] Xue Kai, *Bao ying zui yao* (1555), ed. Xui Ji, *Xue shi yi'an*, *juan* 54, 1–2.

[11] This method can be traced to at least the Tang period (618–907). See Sun Simiao, *Bei ji qian jin yao fang* (652) (Taipei: Taiwan Shang Wu Yin Shu Guan, 1987), *juan* 9, 1. It was called *shi hui fa* (filth-clearing) or *shi kou fa* (mouth-clearing) later in many medical texts. See Wei Yilin, *Shi yi de xiao fang* (1337) (Taipei: Taiwan Shang Wu Yin Shu Guan, 1987), *juan* 11, 9; Zhang Bangtu, *Dou zhen gua* (1550), re-edited by Zhang Taizheng in 1597 (Beijing: Ren Ming Wei Sheng Chu Ban She, 1991), 10–11.

babies from all kinds of disease, smallpox being one of the most important.[12] Nevertheless, others argued that the *tai du* could not be simply removed by this measure after birth.[13] They thought the *tai du* stayed at the *ming men*, and could not be eradicated until such time as it developed into smallpox.

Many physicians assumed that the contaminated matter of *tai du* mainly came from the mother's diet. If the mother was fond of eating acidic, spicy or toxic food, and ate without proper control, the hot *qi* of those toxins would be conveyed to her baby during pregnancy.[14] If the mother was surrounded by heat-inducing circumstances during pregnancy, the various heat toxins would be absorbed by her baby.[15] The more contaminated matter the child absorbed, the more serious the bout of smallpox from which the child suffered.[16] Therefore, the child's condition depended on how much toxin its mother had received.[17]

Some physicians thought that the *tai du* was inherited from the infant's father. In the thirteenth century, Huang Shifeng claimed that the component of the *tai du*, namely *yang du* (male toxin), which originated from the father's *jing* (essence of a male) would decide if the future development of smallpox would take a serious form. The maternal contribution also had *tai du*, namely *yin du* (female toxin), which would develop into sores, scabies, and similar eruptive skin disease.[18] In this case, the effect of the father's *yang du* was more severe than that of the mother's *yin du* and might even be fatal. On the other hand, some physicians thought that the *yin du* which came from the mother would develop into smallpox and the *yang du* which inherited from

---

[12]Xu Chunfu, *You you hui ji* (1556–66). *juan* 88, 848. When the Manchus conquered China, the Imperial Family also applied this method. They gave *fu shou dan* (medicine for longevity) to newborn members to protect them from disease. See Chen Keji ed., *Qing gong yi-an yan jiu* (Beijing: Zhong Yi Gu Ji Chu Ban She, 1990), 313, 320–1, 325, 467.

[13]Yin Youlan, *Dou zhen yi lan* (1564?) (photograph of the Ming edition, Japan, 1965), *juan* 1, 1.

[14]Chen Wenzhong, *Dou zhen fang lun* (1254), cited in *Gu jin tu shu ji cheng yi bu quan lu*, reprint of 1725 edition (Shanghai: Hui Wen Tang Xin Ji Shu Ju, 1937), *juan* 459, 5.

[15]Bai Zhiji ed., *Zeng ding dou zhen ji yao* (1770–1810) (Hing Jing Ge Shu Fang, reprint 1903), *juan* 1, 1.

[16]Liu Xi, *Huo you bian lan* (1510) (original edition), 81.

[17]Yu Tuan, *Yi xue zheng chuan* (1515) (Beijing: Ren Min Wei Sheng Chu Ban She, 1981), 414.

[18]Huang Shifeng, *Mi chuan xiao-er dou zhen yu sui* (1206–1368) (manuscript, Japan, 1770), *juan* 1.

the father would develop into measles.[19] Although physicians held different views on this issue, both hypotheses attempted to explain why smallpox was more serious and fatal than any other disease which had similar symptoms.

Another point of view suggested that the *tai du* was not solely inherited from one of the parents but came from both of them. When the parents conceived their baby, the sexual drive which was thought to contain abundant *yin huo* (lubricious fire) or *hou du* (fire toxin) would produce *tai du* and this was passed on to their child.[20] The temper, desires, the habit of daily life, and diet of the parents before conception would also affect the production of the foetal toxin.[21] For example, if the father enjoyed drinking and taking aphrodisiacs, his *ming men* would become weak, he would accordingly store much heat toxin in his *qi* and this would affect his *jing*. If the mother was impatient and jealous, her *qi* would be disordered and her menses would not come punctually. Then, if she took medicine to warm her womb to improve her health, she would consequently store much heat toxin.[22] If the baby was conceived by drunken parents, it would receive the *tai du* and develop smallpox.[23] In addition, if the parents kept having sexual activity during pregnancy, this would be considered to be contravening the model of the ancient paragons; consequently, the *tai du* which descended to the child would become more severe.[24] These various *tai du* theories suggested that the origin of smallpox had a strong moral connection.

The concept of *tai du* was complex in pre-modern China; physicians did not follow one single theory. No matter whether the *tai du* came from the father, or mother, or both, it was thought to be a necessary condition for developing smallpox. The *tai du* remained quiescent in the *ming men*, like a bean seed just planted into soil, and until the *tai du* was stimulated by ex-

---

[19] Wan Quan, *Wan shi jia chuan dou zhen xin fa* (1549), *Gu jin tu shu ji cheng yi bu quan lu* (1725) edition, *juan* 466, 7–8; Zhu Chungu, *Dou zhen ding lun* (1713) (Gu Su: Qi Xi Tang, 1767), preface; Zhai Liang, *Dou ke hui bian* (1630) (Yin Guangyan edition, 1807), *juan* 1, 1–6. In these texts, we can see the assumption that the *tai du* which came from the mother side would result in smallpox was fairly common, however, the authors disagreed with it.

[20] Zhu Xun, *Dou ke jian* (re-edited by Zhu Fengtai in the Shunzhi period (1644–61), reprint, Japan, 1730), *juan* 1, 1.

[21] Zhu Huiming, *Dou zhen chuan xin lu* (1594) (Shanghai: Qian Qing Tang, 1925), *juan* 1, 1.

[22] Yin Youlan, *Dou zhen yi lan* (1564?) (photograph of the Ming edition, Japan, 1965), *juan* 1, 3.

[23] Zhu Huiming, *Dou zhen chuan xin lu* (1594), *juan* 1, 1.

[24] Yin Youlan, ibid.

ternal factors, it would not sprout and mature.[25] However, there were further requisite elements in order to develop smallpox.

Most physicians believed that the *shi qi* (seasonal vapour) which appeared in disorderly climatic conditions would stimulate the *tai du* of the body, convey it into the pores through the circulation tracts, and then cause it to develop into smallpox.[26] As soon as people were exposed to *shi qi*, it would rapidly enter the body and encounter the *tai du*, triggering it and expelling it out of the *ming men*. Driven by the *shi qi*, the *tai du* dispersed through the blood, and developed into smallpox.

During the thirteenth and fourteenth centuries, physicians in the north of China tended to apply the theory of *wu yun liu qi* (five phases and six *qi*) to smallpox aetiology.[27] The Five Phases, Wood, Fire, Earth, Metal, and Water, together constitute a time cycle equally distributed over the four seasons. The six *qi*, Wind, Cold, Heat, Moist, Dry, and Fire Phases and the Six *qi*, physicians split one of the Phases, Fire, into *jun huo* (ruler-fire) and *xiang huo* (minister-fire). Any abnormal climatic condition could result in physical disorders, for instance, those seasons with excessive *xiang huo* would have many smallpox cases.[28] Therefore, in the theory of the *wu yun liu qi*, climatic conditions with fire factors were thought to be associated with smallpox.

Besides, physicians subsequently thought that every year was composed of different *qi* named *sui qi* (year *qi*), which went through a cycle every sixty years. Each *sui qi* had specific characteristics that would result in people suf-

---

[25] Xue Heshan, "Dou Du Cang Pi Jing Sho", in Tang Lishan ed., *Wu yi hui jiang* (1792) (Shanghai: Ke Xue Ji Shu Chu Ban She, 1983), *juan* 5, 56.

[26] Physicians thought the noxious *shi qi* often happened in the spring. When the winter was warmer than usual, the heat would accumulate and turn to noxious *shi qi* in the next spring. See Pang Anshi (1043–1110?), *Shang han zong bing lun* (Taipei: Taiwan Shang Wu Yin Shu Guan, 1986), *juan* 4, 11–12; Zhu Zhenheng (1281–1358), *You ke quan shu, Gu jin tu shu ji cheng yi bu quan lu* (1725) edition, *juan* 460, 10.

[27] For more details of the theory of *wu yun liu qi* (five phases and six *qi*) in traditional Chinese Medicine, see Paul U. Unschuld, *Medicine in China—A History of Ideas*, (Berkeley: University of California Press, 1985), 170–2; Nathan Sivin, *Traditional Medicine in Contemporary China* (Ann Arbor: University of Michigan, 1987), 70–80, 275–85. However, in premodern China, there were some physicians disagreed with the theory of *wu yun liu qi*. See Yu Tuan, *Yi xue zheng chuan* (1515) (Beijing: Ren Min Wei Sheng Chu Ban She, 1981), *juan* 1, 24.

[28] Zhang Congzheng, *Ru men shi qin* (1228) (Taipei: Taiwan Shang Wu Yin Shu Guan, 1986), *juan* 5, 21–2.

fering from certain diseases, and the diseases would have particular qualities.[29] When the particular *sui qi*, which consisted of heat, interacted with the stored *tai du* of the body, smallpox would burst out.[30] According to this theory, in certain defined years people would tend to be exposed to the *qi* of smallpox, and the symptoms of smallpox sufferers would vary within each of these years.[31] Furthermore, even people who contracted smallpox on different days would have different symptoms.[32] Both concepts of *wu yun liu qi* and *sui qi*, were designed to help the physicians predict the nature, course and outcome of the disease, and prescribe suitable treatments.[33] These two ideas emphasized the importance of the fire factor in smallpox aetiology.

The idea of essential external factors in a case of smallpox was widely accepted in pre-modern China. The conception basically followed the principle of the most authoritative sources of traditional medical doctrines, the *Huang di nei jing* (Inner Canon of the Yellow Emperor),[34] that attributed disease to the heteropathic *qi* (*xie qi*).[35] The human body was thought to be a microcosm, which had to maintain harmony with nature, the macrocosm. If the outer circumstance became disordered, it would necessarily affect the inner aspect. When the smallpox *shi qi* emerged, everyone could be affected except those who had had smallpox. At that time, the vitality of the body would also con-

---

[29] Unknown author, *Dou zhen jing yan liang fang, Gu jin tu shu ji cheng yi bu quan lu* (1725) edition, *juan* 484, 2–4.

[30] Xu Qian, *Ren duan lu* (1644) (Taipei: Taiwan Shang Wu Yin Shu Guan, 1986), *juan* 1, 2–4.

[31] Yin Youlan, *Dou zhen yi lan* (1654?) (photograph of the Ming edition, Japan, 1965), *juan* 1, 10.

[32] Huang Shifeng ed., *Mi chuan xiao-er dou zhen yu sui* (1206–1368) (manuscript, Japan, 1770), *juan* 1.

[33] Meng Jikong, *You you ji* (1510) (Beijing: Zhong Yi Gu Ji Chu Ban She, 1989), *juan* 1, 266–69; Fei Jianzhong, *Jiu pian suo yan* (1659) (Hui Di Tang edition, 1688), *juan* 2, 13–18.

[34] The *Huang di nei jing* was probably written by unknown authors over one century or more and brought together in the first century BC or the early first century AD, *Su wen* (Basic Questions) was an extant part of *Huang di nei jing*. For the date of the *Huang di nei jing*, see Yamada Keiji, "Kotei Naikyo No Seiritsu," *Shiso* 662 (1979): 94–108; David J. Keegan, *The "Huang-Ti Nei-Jing:" the Structure of the Compilation; the Significance of the Structure*, Ph.D. dissertation, University of California, Berkeley, 1988 (Ann Arbor: UMI Reprints, 1991), 13–19; Nathan Sivin, "Huang Ti Nei Ching," in *Early Chinese Texts—A Bibliographical Guide*, ed. Michael Loewe (Berkeley: University of California Press, 1993), 199–201.

[35] Wu Kun annotated (1594), *Nei jing Su Wen wu zhu* (Jinan: Shangdong Ke Xue Ji Shu Chu Ban She, 1984), 15.

tribute to the degree to which the outside influence affected the individual.[36] Hence, *tai du*, *shi qi* and the vitality of the human body together determined the condition of the smallpox victim.

Several other factors could also set off the *tai du*. For example, if children were suddenly frightened, fell down, or became angry, their *tai du* would be easily released.[37] If the child caught *shang han* (cold-damage disorders) or *shang feng* (wind-damage disorders), factors associated with these could also stir the *tai du*.[38] Some physicians asserted that improper diet of children could also stimulate the *tai du*.[39] If the wet nurse ate spicy food, which was considered to contain much heat, her milk would transfer this toxin of heat, *ru du* (milk toxin), to the infant. This *ru du* mixed with its *tai du* and made the smallpox more serious.[40] These external elements were regarded as functioning as catalysts which activated the *tai du*. As one medical text, using an analogy, said, "the process is just like a magnet attracting needles".[41]

As we have seen, the "fire" factor is important in concepts of smallpox aetiology, and this was especially so from the Song Dynasty (960–1279) onward. The ideas of *jun huo* (ruler-fire) and *xiang huo* (minister-fire) are also significant in the internal visceral systems, the five *zang* and six *fu*, of the human body.[42] During the Yuan period, physicians such as Liu Wanshu (1120–1200?), Zhang Congzheng (1156–1228?), Zhang Yuanshu (1151–1234?), and Li Gao (1180–1251), suggested that the symptoms of smallpox were caused by *xiang huo*.[43] According to the *Huang di nei jing*, all symptoms of itchiness, rashes, pain and similar conditions were attributed to the *xinhuo*

---

[36] Zhu Xun, *Dou ke jian* (re-edited by Zhu Fengtai in the Shunzhi period (1644–61), reprint, Japan, 1730), *juan* 1, 3.

[37] Yang Shiying, *Xin kan ren zhai zhi xiao-er fu yi fang lun* (1260) (Taipei: Taiwan Shang Wu Yin Shu Guan, 1986), *juan* 5, 1.

[38] Zhu Zhenheng, *Dan xi xin fa* (1347) (Taipei: Taiwan Shang Wu Yin Shu Guan, 1986), *juan* 5, 61.

[39] Qian Yi, *Xiao-er yao zheng zhi jue* (1093), *Gu jin tu shu ji cheng yi bu quan lu* (1725) edition, *juan* 459, 1.

[40] Zhai Liang, *Dou ke hui bian* (1630) (Yin Guangyan edition, 1807), *juan* 1, 1–4.

[41] Ibid.

[42] For the theory of the visceral systems, the five *zang* and six *fu*, in traditional Chinese medicine, see Nathan Sivin, *Traditional Medicine in Contemporary China* (Ann Arbor: University of Michigan, 1987), 213–36, 349–79.

[43] Liu Wanshu, *Jin Liu Wanshu liu shu, Gu jin tu shu ji cheng yi bu quan lu* (1725) edition, *juan* 459, 10–12; Zhang Congzheng (1156–1228), *Ru men shi qin, juan* 1, 29–32; Zhang Yuanshu (1151–1234?), *Bao min ji* (Taipei: Taiwan Shang Wu Yin Shu Guan, 1986), *juan* 2, 54–55.

(heart-fire).[44] The above physicians and their followers cited above, therefore, believed that the heart visceral system, which corresponded with the Fire Phase, was associated with smallpox. When the *tai du* of the body was stirred by the *shi qi*, the *xiang huo* became active, and sufferers would inevitably have fevers, itchiness, and rashes during the course of smallpox.

Since smallpox was thought to originate from, and be stimulated by, fire factors, those things which were of a "hot" quality would increase the accumulation of the *tai du* and intensify its effects. Therefore, the diet, habits and emotions of the parents would be taken into account. These opinions could be traced from the moral doctrine of the *Huang di nei jing*. According to this text, acidic and strong-flavoured food would incur heat, drunken parents who had sex would store rich heat in the body, and the temper would affect the *qi* and result in disease.[45] Some physicians claimed that they had proven these doctrines by clinical experience. For example, Nei Shangheng, a smallpox physician of the late Ming period (1368–1644), observed that the diet of women did mirror the smallpox situation of their children. He found that those who were fond of mild-flavoured food were prone to deliver children with milder conditions; those who liked rich-flavoured food would have children with more severe and dangerous cases.[46] To these physicians, classical theory and empirical experience combined to put the *tai du* theory on a firm footing.

Yet, the theoretical problems of the *tai du* theory remained. Since physicians claimed that every infant possessed *tai du*, so everyone was a potential smallpox victim. As mentioned earlier, physicians appear to have noticed that the Chinese were not affected by smallpox until their ancestors fought with foreign soldiers sometime around the fourth century AD or earlier;[47] and no reliable record of smallpox was known prior to that time. This obviously raised questions as to why the ancient Chinese had not previously contracted smallpox, and why *tai du* had had no effect on them?[48] In order

[44] *Nei jing Su Wen wu zhu* (Jinan: Shandong Ke Xue Ji Shu Chu Ban She, 1984), 372.

[45] Ibid., 21–2; 165–6; 185.

[46] Nie Shangheng, *Dou zhen huo you xin fa* (1616) (reprinted edition, Japan, 1666), *juan* 1, 1–2.

[47] Smallpox used to be named "lu chuang" (barbarian lesion) because people believed that it was brought into China by soldiers. See Ge Hong, *Zhou hou bei ji fang*, reprint of *Zheng tong dao zang* edition (Shanghai: Shang Wu Yin Shu Guan, 1955), *juan* 2, 235–6.

[48] Zhang Jiebin, *Jing yue quan shu* (1624) (Taipei: Tai Lian Guo Feng Chu Ban She, 1976), *juan* 43, 744; Unknown author, *Dou zhen xin fa yao jue*, ed. Wu Qian, *Yi zong jin jian* (1742) (Beijing: Ren Min Wei Sheng Chu Ban She, 1963), *juan* 56, 7.

to tackle this apparent anomaly, exception was used to prove the rule. One of the essential requirements for achieving a natural life span in the *Huang di nei jing* was to live a proper lifestyle, and any unrestrained indulgence, such as insobriety, debauchery, or overstraining oneself, would harm health.[49] The inference was drawn that the wise ancestors knew how to maintain a balance, so they were able to avoid smallpox. Their descendants, however, had not followed this wise advice, and so more and more people contracted smallpox.[50] Such a comparison with ancient people was seen as providing powerful proof of the effects of lifestyle on smallpox. As mentioned above, their empirical evidence showed that a light diet could alleviate the severity of the smallpox. Through these assumptions, we can see a moral connection between human beings and illness, parents and their children.

A further theoretical problem is that in the Ming and Qing periods (1368–1911), physicians noticed that those who lived beyond the northern borders of China seldom suffered from smallpox.[51] This was another challenge to the *tai du* theory. They therefore adopted a similar strategy to solve this problem, arguing that although the northern peoples had *tai du* in their body, it did not develop into smallpox because they ate less hot food and the climate beyond the north of China was colder, so conditions were not sufficient to set off the disease. Their *tai du* might, however, develop into other diseases.[52] even if they were afflicted by smallpox, the condition was so slight that they were not aware of it.[53] In 1746, some soldiers who came from the northern borders of China passed through central China, and most of them contracted smallpox. They themselves described how when they arrived in China, they were suddenly confronted with hot *qi*, and by which they meant that they felt hot all over.[54] They therefore attributed smallpox to the hot *qi*, which was rare

[49] *Nei jing Su Wen wu zhu* (Jinan: Shandong Ke Xue Ji Shu Chu Ban She, 1984), 1–2

[50] Zhang Jiebin, *Jing yue quan shu* (1624) (Taipei: Tai Lian Guo Feng Chu Ban She, 1976), *juan* 43, 744; Unknown author, *Dou zhen xin fa yao jue*, ed. Wu Qian, *Yi zong jin jian* (1742) (Beijing: Ren Min Wei Sheng Chu Ban She, 1963), *juan* 56, 7.

[51] Zhang Jiebin, *Jing yue quan shu* (1624) (Taipei: Tai Lian Guo Feng Chu Ban She, 1976), *juan* 43, 744.

[52] Nie Shangheng, *Dou zhen huo you xin fa* (1616) (reprinted edition, Japan, 1666), *juan* 1, 1–2. Many paediatric diseases were thought to originate in the prenatal stage in pre-modern China. The *tai du* was one of the major causes. The *tai du* could develop into various diseases, and smallpox was the most serious one. See Yin Youlan, *Dou zhen yi lan* (1564?), *juan* 1, 3.

[53] Nie Shangheng, *Dou zhen huo you xin fa* (1616) (reprinted edition, Japan, 1666), *juan* 1, 1–2.

[54] Shuangwu Zhuren, *Tian hua jing yan* (1813) (oritinal edition, Kui Yuan Tang, 1813), *juan* 1, 1–2.

in their home region. The description, which was recorded in a smallpox text, seemed to fit with the hypothesis that climatic and geographical factors could determine the onset of the disease.

At the time when smallpox was classified as a *shang han* or epidemic disease, the cause of it was simply attributed to the effects of cold in winter, or an unexpected abnormal *qi*.[55] As we have seen, however, from the Five Dynasties and Song period on, smallpox became endemic, children being the main sufferers; in attempting to explain this, physicians surmised that children were full of pure *qi*, so they could be easily affected by abnormal *qi* under any circumstances.[56] However, this assumption was still not sufficient to explain why smallpox was so common and inevitable amongst children, and why smallpox affected people only once in their lifetime. Besides, according to the theory of *shang han* aetiology, children were scarcely affected by cold factors in winter, thus this theory also failed to explain why children often contracted smallpox. In order to deal with these theoretical problems, physicians developed the *tai du* theory. Becoming aware that smallpox was widespread in children, they assumed that the origins of smallpox might exist before birth. Therefore, a link between children and their parents developed, and this connection made everyone a potential victim of smallpox. Smallpox was thought to be inherited, therefore, the *tai du* theory could perfectly explain any individual smallpox case. The *tai du* theory was also applied to explain other child disorders, thus appearance of this theory marks an important stage of the development of paediatrics in pre-modern China.

Qi is a core concept in traditional Chinese medicine. It is regarded as the essential element of nature and the human body, and has to be maintained in balance. The *qi* in nature could affect people in many respects, especially their health. Physicians noticed that in a certain area the condition of smallpox victims was similar at the same time. According to them, this was due to the contagious effects of such *qi*.[57] This idea was felt to be proven by many empirical observations. For instance, Pang Anshi (1043–1110) noted that people

[55] Ge Hong (281–341), *Zhou hou bei ji fang*, reprint of *Zheng tong dao zang* edition (Shanghai: Shang Wu Yin Shu Guan, 1955), *juan* 2, 235–36; Chao Yuanfang, ed., *Zhu bing yuan hou lun* (610), re-edited by Ding Guangdi, (Beijing: Ren Min Wei Sheng Chu Ban She, 1992), *juan* 10, 334–5.

[56] Wang Haogu, *Yi lei yuan rong* (1237), *Gu jin tu shu ji cheng yi bu quan lu* (1725) edition, *juan* 459, 15.

[57] Zhu Zhenheng (1281–1358), *You ke quan shu*, *Gu jin tu shu ji cheng yi bu quan lu* (1725) edition, vol, 460, 1.

often contracted smallpox in spring after a warm winter, and concluded that seasonal *qi* was the cause of this disease.[58] Physicians also cited evidence to support the idea that *shi qi* was of a hot quality, and would influence people in a particular geographical area.[59] The external cause accordingly met the need to interpret any large-scale outbreak of smallpox. On such a basis, the *wu yun liu qi* theory was used to predict the smallpox cycle within years, and, theoretically, people could escape from smallpox by moving to other places before the smallpox *shi qi* arrived.[60]

Physicians also attempted to explain further why individual sufferers in the different places showed varying symptoms and severity of disease while sufferers in many localized epidemics had such similar symptoms. Individual differences of diet, habit, temper, and the degree of *tai du* in the victims were seen as varying. In explaining the condition of an individual smallpox sufferer in this way physicians emphasized that the degree of *tai du* was the most important, while the *shi qi* or other external factors seemed to have less influence. On the other hand, large-scale epidemics of smallpox were seen as being mainly influenced by the *shi qi*, the *tai du* having less effect in such cases; and the victims exposed to *shi qi*, would undergo the same disease process.[61] Some physicians thought that when a certain noxious *shi qi* was rampant, the adult would develop epidemic disease (*wen yi*); in children this would develop into smallpox.[62]

---

[58]Pang Anshi, *Shang han zong bing lun* (Taipei: Taiwan Shang Wu Yin Shu Guan, 1986), *juan* 4, 11–12.

[59]Wan Quan, *Wan shi jia chuan dou zhen xin fa, You ke quan shu, Gu jin tu shu ji cheng yi bu quan lu* (1725) edition, vol, 484, 8–16.

[60]A case is reported on someone who kept moving to escape smallpox for more than forty years and succeeded (Guo Zizhang, *Bo ji xi dou fang lun, Gu jin tu shu ji chen yi bu quan lu* (1725) edition, *juan* 473, 3). Zhu Chungu, a physician who was famous for variolation in the Kangxi period (1682–1713), thought the Mongols did not contract smallpox because of their nomadic way of life, which prevented the *shi qi* from taking effect (Zhu Chungu, *Dou zhen ding lun* (1713) (Gu Su: Qi Xi Tang, 1767), *juan* 2, 1–3). These two cases were used as evidence to prove and enhance the hypothesis of the geographic nature and effect of *shi qi*.

[61]Zhu Zheng, *You ke quan shu, Gu jin tu shu ji cheng yi bu quan lu* (1725) edition, vol, 460, 10; Wan Quan, *Wan shi jia chuan dou zhen xin fa* (1549), *Gu jin tu shu ji cheng yi bu quan lu* (1725) edition, vol, 486, 14–16; Yin Youlan, *Dou zhen yi lan* (1564?) (photograph of the Ming edition, Japan, 1965), *juan* 1, 1–2; Zhai Liang, *Dou ke hui bian* (1630) (Yin Guangyan edition, 1807), *juan* 1, 1–6.

[62]Yin Youlan, ibid., *juan* 1, 1–2.

The Chinese also did not neglect the apparent fact that coming close to the smallpox patient could lead to contracting the disease.[63] Several cases showed that smallpox spread rapidly within a family.[64] Indeed, the Qing Imperial Family used to build isolation shelters in an attempt to prevent from smallpox spreading amongst them.[65] This quarantine activity demonstrated that they were aware of the contagious character of smallpox. Physicians ascribed this contagious phenomenon to the transmission of the smallpox *shi qi*.[66] They assumed that the victim was surrounded with the *shi qi*, so when a person lived with or came into close contact with a sufferer, the *shi qi* would shift onto them, and their condition would be very similar.[67] Either a small-scale or a large-scale outbreak of smallpox could result from this shifting of the *shi qi*. Therefore, in the case of smallpox, the agent of "contagion" is the *shi qi*, contacting with patients may be regarded as an indirect and minor path in pre-modern China.

After the Song Dynasty, the idea that the *tai du* was received from the parents implied that everyone was born with it.[68] The toxin remained in the body until it was excited by external factors, especially the *shi qi*. Only when the *tai du* dispersed, could the body then get rid of the contaminated toxin matter. Since most of the population had undergone this predictable development, people gradually became convinced that contracting smallpox was an inevitable fate. Smallpox was seen as a common event in life, and was considered as a crucial turning-point in determining whether or not a child would grow up successfully.[69] Developing smallpox was thought to be as natural and usual a phenomenon as a snake shedding its skin.[70] It inspired physicians to assert

---

[63] Zhang Gao, *Yi shuo* (Taipei: Taiwan Shang Wu Yin Shu Guan, 1986), *juan* 10, 9.

[64] Wan Quan, *Wan shi jia chuan dou zhen xin fa* (1549), *Gu jin tu shu ji cheng yi bu quan lu* (1725) edition, *juan* 497, 11.

[65] Chang Chia-Feng, "Strategies of Dealing with Smallpox in the Early Qing Imperial Family," in *East Asian Science: Tradition and Beyond*, ed. Hashimoto Keizo, Catherine Jami, and Lowell Skar (Osaka: Kansai University Press, 1995), 199–205.

[66] Zhu Su ed., *Pu ji fang* (1406) (Taipei: Taiwan Shang Wu Yin Shu Guan, 1986), *juan* 402, 1; Guo Zizhang, *Bo ji xi dou fang lun*, *Gu jin tu shu ji cheng yi bu quan lu* (1725) edition, *juan* 473, 3.

[67] Zhu Chungu, *Dou zhen ding lun* (1713) (Gu Su: Qi Xi Tang, 1767), *juan* 2, 21–2.

[68] Xu Qian, *Ren duan lu*, *juan* 1, 2; Fei Jianzhong, *Jiu pian suo yan*, *juan* 1, 5–6.

[69] Zhi Yu Qiao Ke, *Er ke xing* (1723–35?) (Beijing: Zhong Guo Shu Dian, 1987), 42–3.

[70] Wan Quan, *Wan shi jia chuan dou zhen xin fa* (1549), *Gu jin tu shu ji cheng yi bu quan lu* (1725) edition, *juan* 466, 1, 7; Xu Qian, *Ren duan lu* (1644) (Taipei: Taiwan Shang Wu Yin Shu Guan, 1986), *juan* 1, 2.

that smallpox should be allowed to run its course spontaneously,[71] and did not need medical treatment at all.[72] Providing treatment to those with "*shang deng dou*" (first-class smallpox), or "*zhuang yuan dou*" (grade one smallpox) could be dangerous or even fatal.[73] The pox of such cases were seen as normal and good. Those which demanded medical treatment were exceptional types of smallpox, whose pox were considered abnormal in appearance, and which were attributed to various causes, such as having received too much *tai du*, or having disobeyed the restriction of touching any filth or stinking substance in the course of disease.[74] Medical treatment was then applied to try to improve the worst cases by helping the *tai du* disperse smoothly.

Variolation, which gradually became widespread from the Late Ming Dynasty on,[75] is one of the most conspicuous achievements of premodern Chinese medicine. Lymph was collected from patients who had already undergone a successful course of smallpox.[76] After being variolated, those people were supposed to be affected by a *qi* similar to that of the original patient's. Wearing the patient's clothes could also transfer the smallpox *qi* to them.[77] Those who were variolated would have the same symptoms as the previous case. This was felt to ensure that the dispersal of the *tai du* out of the body would be mild, and thus the disease would not be too serious. Variolation cohered with the idea of prevention in traditional Chinese medicine which was regarded as the primary responsibility of the highest type of physician.[78]

---

[71] Shi Jingong, *Dou ke da quan* (1707) (Chi Mu Tang, 1707), *juan* 1, 24–5.

[72] Wang Luan (1405–1524), *You ke lei cui* (Beijing: Zhong Yi Gu Ji Chu Ban She, 1984), *juan* 28, 121; Xu Chunfu, *Dou zhen xie mi, Gu jin tu shu ji cheng yi bu quan lu* (1725) edition, *juan* 474, 5; Shi Jingong, *Dou ke da quan* (1707) (Chi Mu Tang, 1707), *juan* 1, 24–5; Zhuang Yikui, *Dou zheng man jing he bian* (1715?) (prefaced by Bi Wanin, 1799, reprinted in 1848), 26–7.

[73] Zhu Zhenheng, *You ke quan shu, Gu jin tu shu ji cheng yi bu quan lu* (1725) edition, *juan* 460, 10; Zhuang Yikui, ibid.

[74] Wang Kentang, *Zheng zhi zhun sheng* (1597), *Gu jin tu shu ji cheng yi bu quan lu* (1725) edition, *juan* 475, 16–18.

[75] The time during which the Chinese practised variolation remains in debate. See Fan Xingzhun, *Zhong guo yu fang yi xue shi* (Beijing: Ren Min Wei Sheng Chu Ban She, 1953), 110–16; Joseph Needham, *China and the Origins of Immunology*, (Hong Kong: University of Hong Kong, 1980); Donald R. Hopkins, *Princes and Peasants: Smallpox in History*, (Chicago: University of Chicago Press, 1983), 109–10.

[76] Unknown author, *Dou zhen xin fa yao jue*, ed. Wu Qian, *Yi zong jin jian* (1742), *juan* 60, 118.

[77] Some physicians claimed that this method was not very effective. See Unknown author, *Dou zhen xin fa yao jue*, ed., Wu Qian, *Yi zong jin jian* (1742), *juan* 60, 117–18.

[78] *Nei jing Su Wen wu zhu* (Jinan: Shandong Ke Xue Ji Shu Chu Ban She, 1984), 9.

In pre-modern China, the concepts of smallpox aetiology changed in different time frames. From the fourth century to the tenth century, smallpox was mainly classified as *shang han*, or epidemic, or other categories, and it was thought to be caused by cold in winter, or unseasonable *qi*. After the tenth century, smallpox progressively became endemic amongst children, physicians then developed the *tai du* and the *shi qi* theories to explain the origins of smallpox. The *tai du* theory widely applied to other disorders, and was regarded as one of the most important causes of child disease.

In considering the concepts of smallpox aetiology in pre-modern China, we can also see several basic theories embracing a complicate diversity of details. After the tenth century, it was basically believed that smallpox proceeded from two primal causes, the internal cause, *tai du*, and the external cause, *shi qi*. When these two causes coincided in the body, this was sufficient to cause the patient to develop smallpox. This conception of the origin of smallpox was combined with classical medical thought and empirical observation and experience. These theories satisfied the theoretical need of explaining both single and large-scale cases of smallpox.

In general, it was the internal cause, the *tai du*, stored at birth in the *ming men*, that enabled people to have the potential to be affected by smallpox; and, it was the external cause, the *shi qi*, disorderly climatic conditions that brought the abnormal element which led to people developing smallpox by triggering off the dispersal of the *tai du*. The degree of *tai du*, *shi qi*, and the vitality of the body would determine the conditions of the sufferers.

The concept of the *tai du* was complex in pre-modern China. *Tai du* was a contamination inherited from the father, or from the mother, or from both. The origins of the *tai du* was generally thought to be connected with diet, emotions, lifestyle, sexuality, and morality of the parents. The concept of the *shi qi* followed the classical doctrine of traditional Chinese medicine, and attributed disease to heteropathic *qi*. The theories of *wu yun liu qi* and *sui qi* were designed to predict smallpox and to help physicians prescribe treatment. Both internal and external causes of smallpox were associated with fire factors.

People inherited *tai du* before birth, and this element quiescently lodged in the *ming men* was not "contagious" itself. The spread of smallpox was by way of direct contact with the *shi qi*, or by the shifting the *shi qi* from one person to another. *Shi qi* was the medium which made smallpox seem "contagious." This concept of "contagion" in pre-modern China is clearly different from the contemporary understanding of "contagion" in biomedicine.

As soon as the *tai du* had been dispersed, the sufferers safely passed through the most important turning-point of their life. They could not be affected by smallpox any more. The function of the *shi qi* and variolation was to disperse the *tai du* entirely out of the human body. Any medical treatment was simply intended to pull a case of abnormal smallpox back on course.

Since passing the gate of smallpox was regarded as an inevitable process of life, each person would have to confront it. When the *tai du* had been dispersed, the body was purified. Although the course was painful and dangerous, it was believed to be more of a natural development than an unexpected disease.

Key to characters

Chao Yuanfang 巢元方
e'du zhi qi 惡毒之氣
Ge Hong 葛洪
hou 候
huo du 火毒
Huang Di Nei Jing 黃帝內經
jian wu 建武
jing 精
jun huo 君火
Kangxi 康熙
Liu Fang 劉昉
ming men 命門
Pang Anshi 龐安時
qi 氣
re bing 熱病
re du 熱毒
ru du 乳毒
shang deng dou 上等痘
shang feng 傷風
shang han 傷寒
shi hui fa 拭穢法
shi kou fa 拭口法
shi qi 時氣
sui qi 歲氣
Su Wen 素問
tai du 胎毒
wen yi 瘟疫
wu yun liu qi 五運六氣
xiang huo 相火
xie qi 邪氣
yang du 陽毒
yi li bing 疫癘病
yin du 陰毒
yin huo 淫火
zang fu 臟腑
Zhang Gao 張杲
Zhou Hou Bei Ji Fang 肘後備急方
Zhu Bing Yuan Hou Lun 諸病源候論
Zhu Chungu 朱純嘏
zhuang yuan dou 狀元痘

3

THE THREATENING STRANGER: KEWU 客忤 IN PRE-MODERN CHINESE PAEDIATRICS

Christopher Cullen

Introduction

What is *kewu* and why is it worth discussing in the context of a cross-cultural anthology such as this? It is hard to separate the answers to these two questions. Let us take the issue of meaning first. As an initial stratagem we will naturally turn to the definitions to be found in standard dictionaries, including specialist medical glossaries. There is no difficulty in locating a plausible range of meaning for both the characters making up the term we are investigating.

The first is the more common of the two: *ke* normally means "guest" or in a verbal sense "to lodge". In a medical context it refers to some pathogenic factor of external origin lodging in the body as a whole or in some part of it, and hence giving rise to dysfunction of some kind. *Wu* is a rarer word, with senses including "disorder", "reversal", "encroachment". If the meanings of its components were all we had to go on, we would expect the compound *kewu* to indicate a situation in which some alien agency has gained a foothold in the body and caused disorder. As we shall shortly see, this provisional and rough interpretation is confirmed by a more careful analysis.

It seems likely, then, that a discussion of *kewu* will have something to contribute to a comparative intercultural discussion of notions related to contagion. But I think there is more to the problem than this alone. My contention is that by studying texts relating to *kewu* from past and present we can learn something about two interesting problem areas:

(a) The difficulties and dangers of attempting to use modern concepts to interpret texts from distant times and places.

(b) The risks of assuming that a medical text is necessarily good evidence for clinical practice, or indeed good evidence for anything much besides the process by which the text in question was generated—often from other texts.

But let us turn to the texts. A modern Chinese dictionary of Traditional Chinese Medicine (TCM) says, under the heading *xiao'er kewu*:

> Since a child's vital powers are not yet solidly established, if it suddenly sees a strange person, or hears a strange sound, or sees a strange object, this can cause terror and weeping. In extreme cases the face may change colour... and the spleen and stomach may be affected, leading to digestive disorders, including vomiting, diarrhoea and belly pains, accompanied by convulsions [1]

So all we have according to this definition is a scared child with an upset stomach—nothing about contagion here. But modern TCM texts can be very bad guides to medicine in traditional China. So let us go back a couple of thousand years and trace the story from there.

Ke-wu in Early Medical Texts

The most obvious place to look for early references to *kewu* is the *Huangdi neijing* "The inner canon of the Yellow Lord". This composite and varied collection of medical writings probably took something like its present form early in the first millennium AD. In many subsequent centuries it was regarded as an authoritative statement of medical doctrine. Although we frequently find *ke* in the usual technical medical sense mentioned above, *kewu* does not occur as an expression. If we go further back to the texts recovered from the 168 BC burial at Mawangdui, *ke* itself is absent except in its non-technical sense of "a guest". The first explicit use of the term is found in *Jinkui yao lue* "Essentials of the golden casket" a text whose origins lie in the 3rd century AD, where we read:

> *Pills of three ingredients for emergencies*
>
> Rhubarb: 1 ounce; croton bean: 1 ounce; dried ginger: 1 ounce. This drug controls all acute afflictions of the vitals, such as

[1] *Jianming zhongyi cidian*, "A concise dictionary of Chinese medicine," ed. China Academy of Traditional Chinese Medicine (Beijing) (Hong Kong: Joint Publishing Co., 1979), 75–6.

> *zhong e* "struck by evil" or *kewu*, in which the vitals swell up and there is sudden pain like being stabbed with an awl, the breath is hurried, the mouth is clenched shut [*kou jin*], there is corpselike inactivity or sudden death.[2]

There is no suggestion here of a specifically paediatric role for the disease, nor in the next earliest textual instance, which comes from the *Zhouhou beiji fang* "Emergency prescriptions to keep up your sleeve" of Ge Hong (fl. AD 320):

> *Prescriptions for aid in death from sudden* kewu
>
> *Ke-wu* is of the same category as *zhong e* "struck by evil'. [People] mostly get it while on the road or outside the gates. It causes the vitals to knot in pain and swell, and *qi* to beat against the heart and breast. If it is not promptly treated it can actually kill people.[3]

The paediatric connection is first made in the late sixth century compendium *Zhu bing yuanhou zonglun* "On the symptoms and origins of all diseases" by Chao Yuanfang:

> *Symptoms of* zhong kewu *"struck by* kewu*"*:
>
> As for small children being struck by *kewu*, this occurs because their vital powers are weak, so that if they have a sudden encounter with any unusual thing, or with some person they are not used to seeing, they fall ill by becoming encroached upon by daemonic *qi* [*gui shen qi*]. This is called *kewu*. Other names are *zhong ke* "being struck by external [agency]" and *zhong ren* "being struck by a person". The signs are vomiting and purging of a virid, yellow or white colour, with liquid and food particles separated. The belly hurts and the patient arches back in convulsions. The face changes colour. The signs are like those of *xian* "convulsions", but the eyes do not gaze fixedly upwards. The corresponding pulse is thready, hurried and frequent. If treatment is not timely, it will be hard to cure. In cases where a nursing

[2] *Jinkui yao lue*, "Essentials of the golden casket," by Zhang Ji, 3rd century AD, reprinted in Siku quanshu collection, vol. 734 (Shanghai, 1987), 23, 4a–4b.

[3] *Zhouhou beiji fang*, "Emergency prescriptions to keep up your sleeve," by Ge Hong (reprinted in Siku quanshu collection, vol. 734, Shanghai, 1987), 1, 7a.

> mother has overindulged in drink or sex and then suckles the child, [the disorder] is most severe and may be fatal.[4]

But the classic text dealing with this disorder at length is the *Beiji qianjin yaofang* "Essential prescriptions worth a thousand in gold, for emergency use" of Sun Simiao, written around AD 650.[5] Sun was a man whose roles of alchemist, physician, hermit sage and alleged Daoist immortal fitted together well in the times in which he lived, although to a modern reader it is hard to resist the urge to disentangle fact from legend. The subject is evidently a fairly important one for Sun: his heading promises us something substantial:

> Ke wu*: section 4*
>
> [Containing] two discussions, thirty-two prescriptions, one method of moxibustion, two methods of imprecation.[6]

Let us see how this medical compendium describes the symptoms of *kewu*:

> In general, as an illness, *kewu* may be classed as one in which [there is] vomiting and purging of a virid, yellow or white colour, with liquid and food particles separated. The belly hurts and there are convulsions. The face changes colour. The signs are like those of *xian* "convulsions", but the eyes do not gaze fixedly upwards. The corresponding pulse is thready, hurried and frequent.[7]

As this translation suggests, Sun uses almost exactly the same wording as that found in the *Zhu bing yuanhou zonglun*. But when he comes to discuss aetiology we are given a much richer picture;

> The reason why children suffer from *kewu* is that *qi* from persons coming from outside [the home] puffs against them and "encroaches on" (*wu*) them. Another name for this is "being struck by a person" zhong ren. This is *kewu*. [This can happen] even if

---

[4] *Zhu bing yuanhou zonglun*, "On the symptoms and origins of all diseases," by Chao Yuanfang (reprinted in Siku quanshu collection, vol. 734, Shanghai, 1987), 46, 11b.

[5] *Beiji qianjin yaofang*, "Essential prescriptions worth a thousand in gold, for emergency use" by Sun Simiao c. AD 655 (repr. Beijing, 1955).

[6] *Beiji qianjin yaofang*, 5a, 82a.

[7] *Beiji qianjin yaofang*, 5a, 82b.

> it is a member of the family, or it may be someone from a different apartment or another household. [It can happen] even if it is a nursing mother, or if the father or mother return home from outside, where their clothing has passed though the coarse, evil and violent daemonic *qi*, or it may be the *qi* of oxen or horses—all this makes for *kewu*. If while holding [the child] one wheezes breath onto it when the *qi* of the milk has not yet settled, this makes for *kewu* in every case. If the nursing mother undergoes intoxication or sexual excess, her breath is afterwards extremely deleterious to the nursing child, and may be fatal to it. This [danger] cannot but be guarded against.
>
> All who travel by horse will take on the stink of the horse-sweat *qi*. If they do not wash and change their clothing, but go straight back to their children, the child will be struck by "equine *kewu*". If the child suddenly sees a horse coming, or hears a horse neighing in alarm, or if [it comes into contact with] the *qi* of clothing from on the horse, all this will cause the small child to be "struck by equine *kewu*". Guard and protect the child against this. This is especially important for children in their first year of life
>
> [. . .] Whenever an unusual person or anything else comes from outside, that may shock a small child and cause sickness.
>
> If you wish to prevent this, the method is that in all cases where unaccustomed people or anything else comes into the house from outside, you must ensure that the child avoids them and does not catch sight of them. In cases where this cannot be done, burn ox-dung so that the smoke and vapour are always in front of the door. Then all will be well.[8]

Part of what Sun says can be interpreted purely in terms of a warning that children should not be exposed to the unfamiliar. But terms in which he speaks make it hard to avoid reading him as warning of the dangers of some (in our terms) material agency brought into the house by people coming from outside. If so, we would be faced with something that could readily be thought of as contagion in a broad sense. It is worth noting that Sun is careful to distinguish *kewu* from the generality of seasonal childhood ills:

---

[8] *Beiji qianjin yaofang*, 5a, 82a–b.

> There is no season without this disorder. But the fact that small children generally fall ill at the start of autumn is surely not because all small children [are subject to] *kewu*. The reason why children are rarely subject to illness in spring and winter, and are generally ill in autumn and summer is that in autumn and summer childrens' *yang qi* is on the outside. Their vessels are soft and weak. At the start of autumn and the end of summer there is sometimes sudden and extreme cold in the morning and evening. Children being soft and weak on the outside, their *yang* is easily damaged. If sudden and extreme cold breaks the *yang*, the *yang* will become congealed so that there is high fever. If the stomach is cold, there will be diarrhoea. Thus as the end of summer and the beginning of autumn, children generally suffer from fever and diarrhoea. It is not necessarily the case that they are all suffering from *kewu* or [other] daemonic afflictions.[9]

So do we have here a neat distinction between *kewu*, mainly caused by contagion in the broad sense, and disorders of similar symptoms caused by climatic stress? Things are not so simple. Here for instance is a passage which is inserted rather abruptly into the discussion of aetiology cited above, at the point where an omission is marked:

> In the clothes of small children, whether the fabric is of silk or cotton, there must be no hair from the [human] head, and the same goes for their shoes. White clothes and a virid girdle, or virid clothes with a white girdle, all cause "being struck by encroachment" *zhong wu*.[10]

It is hard to see this as anything but a ritual prescription, whose violation will bring disaster. More striking still is the dissonance between any "contagion" interpretation of *kewu* and the following:

> The *Xuan zhong ji* "Record of Mystery" says: In this world there is a female bird, whose name is Guhuo "Aunty Snatcher" (?). Another name is "Daughter of the Heavenly Emperor", or "Secretly Flying Bird", or "Night-Wandering Woman". A further name is

[9] *Beiji qianjin yaofang*, 5a, 82b.
[10] *Beiji qianjin yaofang*, 5a, 82b.

> "Spirit of the Hook-Star". It likes to fly about on dark rainy nights, going to and fro amongst human settlements. This is the creature that can be summoned. This bird is purely female, with no male, and it does not produce [young]. It is produced when *yin qi* is poisonously transformed. It likes to drop hairs and feathers into houses in the midst of people, setting them in the clothes of children. Thereupon this causes the children to suffer from convulsions. When the child falls ill it invariably dies, and then it becomes the young [of this bird]. So when children are below ten years old, their clothes must not be left exposed. This is particularly tabooed in the seventh and eighth months.[11]

We may of course ask ourselves whether or not Sun Simiao or a later editor really intend this passage to be related to *kewu* at all. It may just be that the activities of the bird in question have been seen as relating it to *kewu* through the passage on hairs in clothing quoted above. But this multivalence persists when we look at the question of treatment. Immediately following the description of the symptoms of *kewu* quoted above, we find the following directions:

> One should give Dragon gall (*Gentiana scabra*) Soup as a purge. One may add Ginseng or Angelica in equal quantities with the Dragon gall. When small children are *zhong ke*, quickly look into the mouth to see if to the left and right of the uvula there are green or black swollen nodules as big as a measles pock. They may also be red or white or green. In such as case, one should then quickly use a needle to lance and drain them. One may also scratch them to let [the matter] flow. One may use the head of a hairpin wrapped in cotton to wipe away the blood.[12]

Dragon-gall Soup *longdan tang* has been mentioned by Sun a little earlier (5a, 79a) when it was given as a treatment for the convulsive disorder *xian*, which it will be recalled has similar symptoms to those of *kewu*. But whereas the other treatments for *xian* consist of the administration of classic drug

[11] *Beiji qianjin yaofang*, 5a, 82b. Detailed discussion of the whole question of the mysterious entity referred to here will be found in the study by Yamada Keiji "Ye ming zhi niao" (The bird that calls at night), in *Yamada Gudai dongya zhexue yu keji wenhua* (Philosophy, science and technology in ancient East Asia, Chinese tr.) (Shenyang, 1996), 180–215.

[12] *Beiji qianjin yaofang*, 5a, 82b.

prescriptions or the administration of acumoxa, the same picture by no means emerges when we look at the treatments prescribed for various forms of *kewu* given by Sun (5a, 82b–3b), and listed here in abbreviated form:

1. Fermented bean boluses are made and rubbed over the child's body. On breaking them open fine hairs will be found. Throw the bolus into the road, and pain will cease.
2. Grind silverfish to fragments; place on mother's nipple, or enclose in child's navel, or rub on neck and spine.
3. Plaster mix of stove ash and wormcasts on child's head and other spots.
4. Let child swallow a bean-sized piece of deer-musk
5. Cover child with mother's menstrual cloth.
6. Simmer hair from donkey's front shoulderblade in mother's milk, give child to drink.
7. Ash three inches of mother's girdle and some hair, give child to drink in mother's milk
8. Give saliva from nose of ox.
9. Apply froth from ox's mouth to mother's nipple.
10. Give roasted and pounded rear hanging hoof of pig in mother's milk.
11. Squeeze juice from a horse-dung bolus and give to drink. (This recipe is said to be suitable when the child has been "struck by *kewu*" by some unknown person.)
12. When the stranger responsible for the *kewu* is known, take ten hairs from the top of that person's head, ash with some of the child's girdle, and give to drink in mother's milk.
13. Give the child some wine which has been heated on a bronze mirror.
14. Bathe the child in a heated mixture of horse urine and wine.
15. Bathe the child in pig's urine.
16. Burn moxa at given sites on the child's body, and use a flour paste bolus as in method 1 above. Recite a given imprecation, and throw the bolus into the road.
17. Take a knife and stretch it over the stove. Loosen the child's clothing and jab towards the child with the knife, reciting an imprecation as given. Rub with bolus, split and note presence of hairs, and discard as before.

We note the preoccupation with alien hair and its apparent elimination from the child's body, which is consonant with some of what Sun has already told us about the origins of *kewu*. We note (treatment 12) the attempt to assimilate the alien to the familiar by mingling them. Other treatments seem to be concerned to expel unwanted entities from the body by the use of noxious substances or by threatening gestures. It is hard not to see such actions as demonifuge in intention. The suggested treatments do not fit easily into the mould of classical pharmacotherapy such as that applied to the *xian* disorder, and what is more it is clear that Sun wants us to be careful to distinguish *kewu* from *xian*, as well as from the generality of seasonal illness. Apparently *kewu*, together with its strange aetiology and odd treatments, was as special a case for Sun as it seems to be to a modern reader. But given its special requirements he clearly has no difficulty in prescribing appropriate treatment for it.

Sun goes further than any other early source in giving *kewu* the character of what might be called a "possession disorder". Can it be said that he is an isolated example of this view, or at least that later accounts of *kewu* become less and less "superstitious" as medicine advances? I do not think that this claim can reasonably be made. From the seventh century onwards, Sun's material is copied and echoed in a series of medical compendia, several produced under imperial patronage. There are few signs of any wish to censor the "possession" aspects of the disorder.

Thus still in the Tang dynasty, much of what Sun writes is simply transcribed into the *Wai tai biyao* "Arcane essentials from the Imperial Library", an important work on therapy compiled by Wang Tao (preface AD 752): see chapter 35, p. 37b ff.[13] Under the Song, the great medical encyclopedia *Zhenghe shengji zonglu* "Comprehensive data: a sagely benefaction of the Regnant Harmony reign" (issued AD 1122) discusses *kewu* and related disorders such as *zhong e*, and prescribes classical pharmacological therapies: see chapter 177, 4a–7a. In a later section, however, we read:

> *Ke-wu* is also known as *zu wu* "sudden encroachment". This name refers to the fact that it arrives from the outside, so that it encroaches. It is no different from *zhong e*. It is said that when a person's spirit and vitality is weak, then daemonic, fierce and poisonous *qi* is able to encroach [... symptoms are described ...]

[13] *Wai tai biyao*, "Arcane essentials from the Imperial Library," by Wang Tao (reprinted in Siku quanshu collection, vol. 737, Shanghai, 1987).

> In such cases one always has resort to the methods of amulets and imprecations.[14]

Several different imprecatory texts and rituals then follow, after which we are given drawings of various amulets. The two given on page 4b are said to be particularly effective against *kewu*; they are immediately preceded by the two imprecations given by Sun Simiao. Another collection of material on *kewu* is to be found in a paediatric compendium first printed in AD 1150 by Liu Fang, *You you xin shu* "A new treatise on the proper treatment of the young".[15] The subdivisions of the topic given by Liu are somewhat are more detailed than those in Sun's account, but most of his treatments (including imprecations) are to be found there, together with many methods from other authors. It does not seem that medical writers under the Song felt any more doubt about the nature of *kewu* than did their Tang predecessors, nor did they experience any problems about continuing to record demonifuge treatments.

The story could be continued through a number of later medical sources. These would include, for instance, the fifth volume of Wang Kentang's influential *Liu ke zhunsheng* "Standards for the six specialties" (preface AD 1607), in which he deals with paediatrics.[16] Chapter 9, pages 783–6 contain much material that we have already discussed. But there is little point in going over such sources in detail. The main point is well established that *kewu* persists as a category of disorder through the centuries, retains its essential aetiology of encroachment/possession, and never seems to be in any danger of being dropped as a result of any criticism based on its demonological origins. Even when we come to the writing of an eighteenth-century physician like Chen Fuzheng, who takes a decidedly critical attitude towards earlier medical thinking, the category of *kewu* is retained. In his *You you jicheng* "Compendium on the proper treatment of the young" (printed AD 1750) he begins in familiar terms:

> *Ke-wu* in children originates from the fact that the child's prenatal endowment is insufficient, and its vital powers are not yet at their full, so that noxious alien *qi* from without is able to take

[14] *Zhenghe shengji zonglu*, "Comprehensive data: a sagely benefaction of the Regnant Harmony reign," (issued 1122, reprinted Taipei, 1978), 196, 1a.

[15] *You you xin shu*, "A new treatise on the proper treatment of the young," by Liu Fang (1150, reprinted Beijing, 1981), chapter 7, 196–7.

[16] *Liu ke zhunsheng*, "Standards for the six specialties," by Wang Kentang (reprinted Taipei, 1979).

> advantage of the situation. [...] This may take place when a stranger appears, or when some animal suddenly bursts in upon the child, or when someone playfully rides on an ox or horse when holding the child, or when the father or mother comes back home on horseback after a long journey, and holds the child before their clothes have been steamed, so that the horse sweat and improper *qi* enters through the child's nose.[17]

Chen goes on to suggest the need for a new concept of *neiyin kewu* "endogenous *kewu*" stemming from frustration of the child's wishes because of its inability to express itself. After suggesting a variety of conventional pharmacological remedies, he goes on to discuss *zhong e* "being struck by evil".

This is like *kewu* but is more severe. *Kewu* is in every case due to the improper *qi* of people or animals from outside [the child's normal environment], but in the case of *zhong e* the child is struck by evil and poisonous *qi*, such as that from rotting corpses in old coffins, old trees in sinister shrines, dry wells in chilly temples, ruined houses or dark ditches—all of them have evil and poisonous *qi* in them, and if the child encounters it, it will enter through the nose. (*You you jicheng* 2, 140.)

One cannot help noticing that even here the sources of the encroaching *qi* listed by this literate and rationalistic physician are just the kind of places where folk belief would expect a child to run the risk of demonic possession. Sun Simiao would have agreed with the risk assessment, even if he might have been less restrained in his description.

It seems, therefore, that we have in the case of *kewu* a clear example of the language of possession remaining in use in élite Chinese medicine for many centuries, with the concept itself being at best only lightly veiled under rationalistic forms of words. But things may not be as simple as that.

The point to observe is that all our examples so far have been taken from a limited range of medical literature, which is principally concerned with listing disorders more or less exhaustively, and in most cases following each disorder described with a long list of possible therapies. We cannot assume that the balance of attention paid to either disorders or therapies in such works is a close approximation to what would be found from observation of the actual clinical practice of Chinese physicians. Now of course it would be quite unreasonable to expect to find any such dispassionate reporting of practice in

[17] *You you jicheng*, "Compendium on the proper treatment of the young," by Chen Fuzheng (1750, reprinted Beijing, 1988), 2, 138.

the medical literature, written as it is to serve the diverse personal agendas of the physicians who generated it. Nevertheless, in the so-called *yi'sn* genre, which is found from the sixteenth century in increasing quantity, we do have collections of physicians' cases, sometimes compiled by themselves but more usually by their disciples. While the purpose of these is clearly to enhance the reputation of the physician involved and to promulgate his views, we do at least have the chance of seeing whether or not *kewu* appears in a kind of medical writing with possibly closer links to practice than the kinds of book we have so far considered.

The answer is decidedly negative. Inspection of a number of standard collections of cases largely fails to reveal the use of *kewu* as an ordering category in those cases in which physicians are treating children. In one instance found in a late Qing collection, a Ming dynasty physician says of a disorder caused by a pregnant woman picking up a child in her arms that is "a similar sort of thing to *kewu* [*ru kewu shi lei*]".[18]

It is of course hard to prove the negative proposition that *kewu* was never used as the name of a disorder actually met in treatment. The nearest I can get is to cite one instance in which *kewu* might have been expected, but we get something else instead. The example comes from the collected cases of the sixteenth-century physician Wang Ji. In this instance he is describing the illness that befell his own grandson:

> When he was not yet a month old his nurse took him out wrapped up in her bosom, and went to watch some spring festivities. At that time the wind was cold and cutting. When they came home, he cried and would not suckle, and he had Fright convulsions from time to time. [...] I said: "When a child is new-born, its vital powers are not yet sufficient. Wind and cold can easily attack, and in this case it must be that noxious wind has taken advantage of the child's depleted state to enter....[19]

The disorder named as Fright convulsions, *jing xian* is one very commonly met in the theory and practice of paediatrics. I have discussed its links with folk beliefs elsewhere.[20] It seems that for all practical purposes physicians (or

[18] *Xu mingyi lei'an*, "Case records of illustrious physicians extended," edited by Wei Zhixiu (1770, reprinted Taipei, 1971), 34, 792a.

[19] *Shishan yi'an*, "Stone Mountain Case Histories," by Wang Ji, compiled by his disciple Chen Jue, (1531, reprinted in Siku quanshu collection, vol. 765, Shanghai, 1987), 2, 42a–b.

[20] "Patients and Healers in Late Imperial China" *History of Science* 31(2): 99–150).

at least those represented in the *yi'an* literature) faced with children attacked by powerful external influences preferred to use the language of Fright to that of possession and contagion implicit in the concept of *kewu*. Despite this, the concept of *kewu* continued to hold its place in the descriptive literature. While we would evidently be well advised not to be surprised at the persistence of non-rationalistic discourse in certain contexts, it does seem that we would be equally well advised to learn the lesson that there is not a single medical literature in China, but several, each of which needs to be treated on its own terms. Whether or not we feel we can find ideas corresponding to contagion in Chinese will evidently depend very much on where we are prepared to look.

Key to characters

Beiji qianjin yaofang 備急千金要方
Chao yuanfang 巢元方
Chen Fuzheng 陳復正
Chen Jue 陳桷
Ge Hong 葛洪
Gu huo 姑獲
gui shen qi 鬼神氣
Huangdi neijing 黄帝內經
Jianming zhongyi cidian 簡明中醫辭典
jing xian 驚癇
Jinkui yao lue 金匱要略
ke 客
ke-wu 客忤
kou jin 口噤
Liu Fang 劉昉
Liu ke zhunsheng 六科準繩
longdan tang 龍膽湯
Mawangdui 馬王堆
neiyin ke-wu 內因客忤
qi 氣
ru ke-wu zhi lei 如客忤之類
Shishan yi'an 石山醫案
Sun Simiao 孫思邈
Wai tai biyao 外臺秘要
Wang Ji 汪機
Wang Kentang 王肯唐
Wang Tao 王濤
Wei Zhixiu 魏之琇
Wu 忤
xian 癇
xiao'er ke-wu 小兒客忤
Xu mingyi lei'an 續名醫類案
Xuan zhong ji 玄中記
yi'sn 醫案
You you jicheng 幼幼集成
You you xin shu 幼幼新書
Zhang Ji 張機
Zhenghe shengji zonglu 政和聖濟總錄
zhong e 中惡
zhong ke 中客
zhong ke-wu 中客忤
zhong ren 中人
Zhouhou beiji fang 肘後備急方

Zhu bing yuanhou zonglun 諸病源候總論 zu wu 卒忤

Part II

INDIA

4

NOTIONS OF "CONTAGION" IN CLASSICAL INDIAN MEDICAL TEXTS

Rahul Peter Das

1. According to modern English dictionaries, *contagion* in a medical context refers to the transference of disease[1] by contact. When we seek to examine the notions pertaining to such contagion in ancient India, it seems to stand to reason that we should expect relevant information to be present especially in texts dealing for the most part with matters of a medical nature, i.e., Āyurvedic texts. When we however turn to such texts, we discover to our surprise that contagion seems to play only a minor role in them.

2. This does not of course mean that nothing relevant at all is mentioned or discussed. Indeed, what seems a very clear example is found in *Aṣṭāṅgahṛdaya.*, Ni 14.41 f = *Aṣṭāṅgasaṃgraha*, Ni 14(page 73b), which says:

> "Through touch, [and] through indulgence in eating, sleeping etc. together, all diseases (*gadāḥ sarve*) commonly/for the most part (*prāyaśas*) are such as pass from one to another (*sañcārin-*), especially disorders of the eye and the skin."[2]

I am grateful to Harunaga Isaacson for commenting on an earlier version of this study.

[1] I have stuck to the term "disease" in this essay for reasons of practicality, and not in an effort to prejudice the discussion on the actual meanings and correct applicability of the terms "disease", "illness" and "sickness". On this problem see e.g., Robert A. Hahn, "Rethinking 'Illness' and 'Disease'," in *South Asian Systems of Healing*, ed. E. Valentine Daniel and Judy F. Pugh, Contributions to Asian Studies 18 (Leiden: E. J. Brill, 1984), 1–23, and Ronald Kaiser, *Die Professionalisierung der ayurvedischen Medizin und deren Rolle im indischen Medizinpluralismus*, Kölner Ethnologische Arbeitspapiere 3 (Bonn: Holos Verlag, 1992), 143 (with further references). On the relevant Sanskrit nomenclature see also G. J. Meulenbeld, *The Mādhavanidāna and its Chief Commentary. Chapter 1–10. Introduction, Translation and Notes*, Orientalia Rheno-Traiectina 19 (Leiden: E. J. Brill, 1974), 505.

[2] *sparśaikāhāraśayyādisevanāt prāyaśo gadāḥ*
sarve sañcāriṇo netratvagvikārā viśeṣataḥ.

Here *sañcārin-* "moving together/around/over to", in the sense of "passing from one to another" or "transmitted", seems to refer to the means of transmission we usually have in mind when speaking of contagion. One is even inclined to render *sañcārin-* as "contagious"; however, since the text expressly mentions either all diseases or almost all diseases (depending on how we translate *prāyaśas*), we cannot take it to refer specifically to contagious, or maybe infectious, diseases without at the same time supposing that all or almost all diseases were considered contagious or infectious, in which case it does not make sense any more to stick to our modern distinction of contagious and non-contagious, or infectious and non-infectious, diseases.

3. We clearly have a problem here. Trying to shed some light on the matter, I examined occurrences of the verb *sam*$\sqrt{}$*car* "move together/around/over to" and its derivatives in Indian medical texts. As within the framework of this small study it was not possible to go through a large mass of texts, I had to limit myself to the so-called "classical" texts *Aṣṭāṅgahṛdayasaṃhitā*, *Aṣṭāṅgasaṅgraha*, *Carakasaṃhitā* and *Suśrutasaṃhitā*; whether my findings are applicable to other medical texts too will have to be examined separately, in which connection we might also have to distinguish between older and later texts. But be that as it may, amongst all the relevant passages with forms of *sam*$\sqrt{}$*car* or its derivatives,[3] I found only one which referred to something similar to the passage just quoted; all the others referred to other matters. The solitary passage I did find is *Aṣṭāṅgasaṃgraha*, Śā 1(275a), which tells us that a man should wed a woman from a family which does not have *sañcārin-* diseases. Does this refer to diseases transferred by contagion, or do we rather have a reference to hereditary diseases here? The commentator Indu gives as examples the diseases *kuṣṭha-* and *paiṅgalya-*. The latter refers to a yellowish or reddish brown colouration, which makes it difficult to find out what exactly Indu means. The former term, *kuṣṭha-*, is a name applied to various skin diseases, seemingly including several forms of leprosy, but not synonymous with "leprosy".[4] According to *Suśruta.*, Ni 5.28 *kuṣṭha-* is sure to arise in the child of

---

[3] *Aṣṭāṅgahṛdaya.*, Sū 22.11$\frac{1}{2}$; 23.26; 29.6, Śā 1.62, Ni 14.42; 16.35, Ci 7.80, Ut 1.36; 17.3; 21.58, *Aṣṭāṅgasaṃgraha*, Sū 21(page 160b); 27(208b); 31(233b); 31(234a); 32(238b); 34(243b); 35(249a), Śā 1(275a), Ni 14(73b); 16(81b), Ci 9(173b); 24(303a), Ut 1(10b); 21(150a); 22(163a); 25(182a); 35(266b), *Caraka.*, Sū 11.9–10, Śā 1.70; 1.106, Ci 21.30; 28.65, *Suśruta.*, Sū 15.11; 17.5; 18.27; 21.27; 29.49, Ni 1.13; 1.30, Śā 1.16; 7.14, Ci 37.87; 40.62, Ut 6.25; 42.4. This list does not take into account occurrences found in variant readings (including those mentioned by commentators).

[4] For details see e.g., R. E. Emmerick, "Some Remarks on the History of Leprosy in India," *Indologica Taurinensia* 12 (1984): 93–105, and *Idem*, "Die Lepra in Indien," in *Aussatz · Lepra*

parents affected by it, i.e., to be hereditary.[5] Should therefore *sañcārin-* indeed refer to hereditary diseases here, then we would have the same term being applied at two different places in *Aṣṭāṅgasaṃgraha* to diseases which we today regard as having different modes of transmission. From this it would seem to follow that not the mode of transmission, but the fact of transmission itself was what led to the characterization of diseases as *sañcārin-*.

4. However, we do not know whether Indu is right in his explanation. Matters become even more complicated when we consider *Suśruta.*, Ni 5.33 f, which, only shortly after the passage (5.28) in which *kuṣṭha-* has been called a hereditary disease, states:

> "Through connection/intercourse[6] (*prasaṅga-*), bodily contact, breath, eating together, and also lying and sitting together, [and using the same] clothes, garlands and unguents, *kuṣṭha-* and fever, and desiccation (consumption?) (*śoṣa-*), and running of the eyes indeed, and diseases 'added on' pass on/over/through (*saṅkrāmanti*) from man to man."[7]

The description of this verse rules out hereditary diseases, so that the two *Suśruta.* passages too, in the way they describe how one can be affected by *kuṣṭha-*, ultimately lead to the same sort of difficulty as the use of *sañcārin-* in two different passages of *Aṣṭāṅgasaṃgraha* does. In this case too, therefore, a difference between what we would call hereditary and contagious diseases does not seem to have been made.

5. But there is even more to come. What has been translated as "added on" here is in the original *aupasargika-*, the adjectival derivation from *upasarga-*, whose basic, neutral meaning seems to be "adding on, addition", as evinced too by the meaning of the verb *upa√sṛj*: "let loose towards" (in various connotations) → "add on". Thus it would seem plausible to assume that in the passage above *aupasargika-* has been used to characterize diseases "passed on".

· *Hansen-Krankheit. Ein Menschheitsproblem im Wandel. Teil II: Aufsätze*, ed. Jörn Henning Wolf (Würzburg: Deutsches Aussätzigen-Hilfswerk, 1986), 185–99.

[5]On this cf. also Emmerick (1986), 193.

[6]Not in the narrow sexual sense.

[7]*prasaṅgād gātrasaṃsparśān niśvāsāt sahabhojanāt*
sahaśayyāsanāc cāpi vastramālyānulepanāt
kuṣṭhaṃ jvaraś ca śoṣaś ca netrābhiṣyanda eva ca
aupasargikarogāś ca saṅkrāmanti narān naram.

If we had only this passage, then we might understand *aupasargika-* as "contacted" and hence "contagious", but in the light of what has just been pointed out we must reckon with the possibility of this assumption being far too facile. In other words, we must ask what exactly or at least approximately is meant by *aupasargika-*.

6. Moreover, the exact nature of what is thus passed along is not clear—is it the disease itself, or is it something bringing this forth? That this is quite a problem is demonstrated by a native source commenting on the passage given last. We find *Suśruta.*, Ni 5.33 f incorporated in a later work, *Mādhava-nidāna* 49.42 f, and the still later commentary (called *Madhukośa*) on this work remarks on this passage:

> "*aupasargika-* [diseases] [means] *pāpa-* diseases etc. and those originating from the *upasarga-* of evil spirits (*bhūta-*). *saṅkrāmanti* (i.e.: pass on/over/through) [means] enter/take possession of/ reach (*āviśanti*).[8] And the passing on/over/through (*saṅkrānti-*) of diseases is to be understood as [happening] in the case of contact/connection/association (*saṃsarga-*) with persons characterized by *pāpa-* (*pāpin-*), [namely] those with *kuṣṭha-*[9] etc., due to a *pāpa-* (adjective) passing on/over/through (*saṅkrānti-*) (or: due to the passing on/over/through of *pāpa-*), or because of the power/faculty of (or: or as a consequence of/through) (*prabhāvāt*) morbid change (*vikāra-*)."[10]

An alternative translation of the last part is:

> "And the passing on/over/through of diseases is to be understood as [happening] in the case of contact/connection/association with persons characterized by *pāpa-*, [namely] those with *kuṣṭha-* etc., or because of the power/faculty of (or: or as a consequence of/through) morbid change due to a *pāpa-* (adjective) passing on/over/through (or: due to the passing on/over/through of *pāpa-*)."

---

[8] This explanation of *saṅkrāmanti* is also offered by Ḍalhaṇa in his commentary on *Suśruta.*, Ni 5.33 f.

[9] Cf. note 4.

[10] *aupasargikāḥ pāparogādayo bhūtopasargajāś ca. saṅkrāmanty āviśanti. rogasaṅkrāntiś ca kuṣṭhiprabhṛtipāpijanasaṃsarge pāpasaṅkrānter vikāraprabhāvād vā boddhavyā.*

7. The term *pāpa-* is often translated as "sin(ful)", but such a meaning is clearly not adequate in the given context. Now in late Vedic texts, *pāpa-* as an adjective means "bad", and can as such also be substantivized; it refers to something harmful, condemnable or unwanted, and in its substantivized form is more often than not used to denote a might which we today would call supernatural.[11] An active might be in keeping with the use of *saṅkrāmanti* and *saṅkrānti-* (from the verb *sam√kram*) in the passage above; however, this neglects possible metaphoric usage similar to that in English, so that we must be careful in our deductions from the passage quoted. On the other hand, it does seem as if, at least in the eyes of a traditional exegete (about nine hundred years before our time) of the *Suśruta.* passage, the processes alluded to here are such as would—at least in part—be termed supernatural by us.

8. To check the validity of this deduction, I examined other occurrences of *upa√sṛj* and its derivatives in Indian medical texts. In this, I had to limit myself in the same way as in my examination of *sam√car* and its derivatives. But even with this limitation, I was unable to examine in detail all occurrences of the terms mentioned,[12] as this would have taken me far beyond the scope of this study. Indeed, in many cases it will take extensive in-depth research to say exactly what the terms mentioned mean, or the answer may even be unavailable.

9. Nevertheless, my cursory study did turn up some interesting facts. The verb *upa√sṛj*, not confined to a use with diseases alone, seems in many cases to mean simply "afflict" or the like, and its derivatives thus something similar (e.g., "affliction"). In some cases an even more neutral meaning "joined with" or the like (with similar derivatory meanings) seems to be in place. On the other hand, *aupasargika-* is clearly defined as referring to superinduced

---

[11] Some years ago I wrote a book-length study on this ("*pāpá* und *pāpmán* im Śatapathabrāhmaṇa"), which I have not yet published, but plan to do some time after suitable revision. Since this study has copious bibliographic information, I beg my readers to bear with me if for now I refrain from quoting relevant literature.

[12] *Aṣṭāṅgahṛdaya.*, Ni 5.46; 5.57, Ci 6.82, Ut 12.32; 21.7, *Aṣṭāṅgasaṃgraha*, Sū 3(page 22a); 25(189b); 28(212a); 36(252a), Śā 1(278b); 4(309b), Ni 5(36b); 5(37b); 10(53a), Ci 8(163a), Ka 1(314b); 1(315a); 1(318a); 3(331a), Ut 6(56b); 9(73a); 15(113a); 25(175b); 49(417b); 49(429a), *Caraka.*, Sū 1.98; 12.8; 13.71; 19.4,4; 20.4; 25.5, Ni 1.23; 4.9; 7.4; 8.4, Vi 1.25.4–5; 3.7,3; 5.7; 8.5, Śā 5.12; 8.6; 8.55; 8.60, Ci 12.5; 17.7; 17.48; 21.42; 22.7; 22.17; 25.120, Ka 1.21; 1.24; 1.26; 12.43; Si 1.34; 8.16; 9.6; 9.8, *Suśruta.*, Sū 1.8,4; 1.14; 13.5–7; 24.7; 34.15; 35.18; 45.11; Ni 5.34; 6.24; 12.7; 13.48; 13.52; 16.9, Śā 2.5; 8.5; 10.46; 10.50–51; 10.56, Ci 2.96; 27.10; 33.12; 35.21, Ka 1.75, Ut 1.6; 7.41; 24.24; 28.3; 37.21; 40.20; 43.11; 43.15; 45.9; 65.18. This list does not take into account occurrences found in variant readings (including those mentioned by commentators).

diseases (i.e., diseases "added on" to others) in *Suśruta.*, Sū 35.18,[13] and this usage of *upa√sṛj* or its derivatives is also found in other passages. Obviously, there is some potential for confusion here, and that I am not the only one to have this feeling is made evident by the remark of the commentator Toḍaramalla on *upasarga-* in *Aṣṭāṅgahṛdaya.*, Ni 5.46: this may, he says, refer to a superinduced disease, or, alternatively, to a disease in general[14] (by contrast, the commentaries of Śrīdāsa on this passage in *Aṣṭāṅgahṛdaya.*[1] and Indu on the identical passage *Aṣṭāṅgasaṃgraha*, Ni 5(36b) take *upasarga-* to refer to a superinduced disease only).

10. Yet in spite of these terminological difficulties it does seem as if we were on the right track in holding that *upa√sṛj* and its derivatives can refer to some sort of transference too, though maybe only sporadically. Thus *Caraka.*, Sū 20.4, explaining what are clearly endogenous (*nija-*) and exogenous (*āgantu-*) diseases, gives disorders of the morbific entities[15] as the reason for the former, whereas the latter appear, according to the text, due to various external injuries, bewitchment, curses, evil spirits (*bhūta-*) and *upasarga-*.[16] Even though the last two terms follow one upon the other, the fact that what to us are natural and supernatural causes are mentioned mixed up with each other seems to show that this is of no importance; in other words, *upasarga-* can still well be what is to us something stemming from 'natural' causes. In any case, it afflicts the body from without. This mode of affliction is also presupposed by Indu, who in his commentary on *Aṣṭāṅgasaṃgraha*, Ut 15(113a) explains *aupasargika-* of the text as *āgantuka-* "exogenous".

11. But the classification of diseases in Indian medical texts is quite problematic—and has unfortunately not been studied in any sort of detail yet.[17] That this is relevant for us too is borne out by *Suśruta.*, Ut 1.6,

---

[13] "*aupasargika-* by name is the disease which, produced at a later time, adds [itself] (*upasṛjati*) to a disease arisen before" (*aupasargiko nāma yaḥ pūrvotpannaṃ vyādhiṃ jaghanyakālajāto vyādhir upasṛjati*); on *upasṛjati* the commentator Ḍalhaṇa rightly remarks: *samīpa ātmānaṃ nayati* "leads itself to the vicinity".

[14] *upasargād anyarogābhiṣaṅgāj jvarādirogadīrghakālānubandhāt. athavopasargād iti rogāt. upasargaśabdaḥ sāmānyena rogamātre 'pi vartate.* This remark from the hitherto unpublished commentary has been given by the editor in a footnote.

[15] These are usually called "humours" in the secondary literature.

[16] *mukhāni tu khalv āgantor nakhadaśanapatanābhicārābhiśāpābhiṣaṅgābhighātavyadhabandhanaveṣṭanapīḍanarajjudahanaśastrāśanibhūtopasargādīni. nijasya tu mukhaṃ vātapittaśleṣmaṇāṃ vaiṣamyam.*

[17] There seem to be various, and often conflicting, classifications. For some relevant material see the discussion and references on 132 ff., particularly 144 ff., of Albrecht Wezler, "On Two

where disorders which are "*upasarga-* etc." (*upasargādi-*) and those which are *āgantu-* are differentiated, which is at variance with *Caraka.*, Sū 20.4 if *āgantu-* should mean the same here, this being, however, admittedly not certain in the absence of other relevant information. The commentator Ḍalhaṇa explains "*upasarga-* etc." as "fever etc.", and *āgantu-* in the given context as "derangement etc." (*unmādādi-*). In doing so, he obviously seeks a connection with *aupasargika-* in *Suśruta.*, Ni 5.33 f cited above. But he also clearly sees problems, for he goes on to say:

> "Now it may be said: because of the causation of derangement etc. through evil spirits, how can there be *āgantu*-hood (or: because of the causation through evil spirits, how can there be *āgantu*-hood of derangement etc.)? Because the *āgantu-* ones are caused by beating etc. It is true: because of external causation of derangement etc. there is *āgantu*-hood (or: because of external causation there is *āgantu*-hood of derangement etc.). Gayin[18] however explains: '*upasarga-* etc. [means] non-human *upasarga-* etc. And they, [i.e.] epilepsy (*apasmāra-*) and derangement, are explained in [the chapters on] the knowledge of evil spirits (*bhūtavidyā-*).[19] It is they which are *āgantu-*.' "[20]

12. I have tried to translate this passage as literally as possible to make its difficulties clear. Maybe it is corrupt, or maybe I have not grasped its import fully. But be that as it may, at the very least it does appear as if *upasarga-* and what it is connected or contrasted with caused difficulties to the commentators. And one thing must strike one especially, namely that Ḍalhaṇa has difficulties in reconciling an in our eyes supernatural cause with *āgantu-*. Might

Medical Verses in the Yuktidīpikā, " *Journal of the European Āyurvedic Society* 1 (1990): 127–48, and also Reinhold F. G. Müller, "Krankheitsbeurteilungen als ≪constitutional≫ und ≪accidental≫ in der indischen Medizin," *Gesnerus* 21 (1964): 212–15, and *Idem*, "Az ősi indiai seborvosok hétcsoportos betegségfelosztása—kritikai ismertetés," and "Beurteilung einer Siebengliederung von Krankheiten durch indische Wundärzte," *Communicationes ex Bibliotheca Historiae Medicae Hungarica* 32 (1964): 9–18 and 19–29. Note too *Madanamahārṇava* 5(63).

[18] = Gayadāsa, whose commentary on this portion of *Suśruta.* has not been found.

[19] According to traditional classification, the Āyurveda is divided into eight different branches, one of these being *bhūtavidyā-*.

[20] *nanu bhūtanimittatvād unmādādīnāṃ katham āgantukatvam. yataḥ prahārādikṛtā āgantavaḥ. satyam. bāhyanimittatvād unmādādīnām āgantukatvam. gayī tūpasargādayo 'mānuṣopasargādayaḥ. te cāpasmāronmādā bhūtavidyābhihitāḥ. ta evāgantava iti vyākhyānayati.*

we conclude from this that according to him it would rather fit the opposite of *āgantu-*, namely *upasarga-*? But we cannot be sure whether this is indeed Ḍalhaṇa's problem; for all we know it might be something quite different, so that it is probably best not to dwell too long on this point, at least not until more material on Ḍalhaṇa's problem is available. However, Gayin/Gayadāsa expressly connects *upasarga-* with something to us supernatural, though in the end he seems to equate *upasarga-* and *āgantu-* too, maybe with passages such as *Caraka.*, Sū 20.4 in mind (or maybe he read the *Suśruta.* passage differently).

13. All this does seem to show a connection here between *upa√sṛj* and its derivatives and something that to us moderns would be supernatural. This is even more so when one considers *Suśruta.*, Sū 24.7. In this passage, diseases originating through divine power (*daivabalapravṛtta-*) are explained, and together with hostility towards gods, curses and sorcery we find diseases arisen due to *upasarga-* mentioned.[21] The latter are explained by Ḍalhaṇa as fever etc. arisen due to the vicinity of diseased persons.[22] If this is correct, then we have here a clear divine or at least supra-human connection with what we would consider to be contagion, and that is something difficult for us to comprehend. Matters are not made easier by what follows. The *Suśruta.* passage goes on to say that all these diseases are twofold according to whether they are caused by lightning or thunder, or by flesh-eating demons (*piśāca-*) etc., and twofold again according to whether they are caused by contact/connection/association (*saṃsarga-*) or are sudden/accidental (*ākasmika-*).[23] Explaining the difference between *upasarga-* and *saṃsarga-*, Ḍalhaṇa says that the former refers to association/contact (*samparka-*) with those having fever or other diseases, whereas the latter refers to association/contact with those hostile to gods and the like.[24] Whatever the terms employed here may actually signify, from this it at the very least follows that there existed theories on the transmission of diseases through contact encompassing more than what is associated with the term *contagion* in modern usage.

[21] *daivabalapravṛttā* (misprinted *daivabalapravṛtā*) *ye devadrohād abhiśaptakā* (variant: *abhiśastakā*) *atharvaṇakṛtā upasargajāś ca.*

[22] *upasargajā iti upasṛjyanta ity upasargāḥ pīḍitajanasamīpotpannā jvarādayaḥ.*

[23] *te 'pi dvividhā vidyudaśanikṛtāḥ piśācādikṛtāś ca. punaś ca dvividhāḥ saṃsargajā ākasmikāś ca.*

[24] *upasargajasaṃsargajayor ayaṃ viśeṣaḥ. upasargajā jvarādirogapīḍitajanasamparkād bhavanti. saṃsargajāś ca devādidrohakajanasamparkād bhavanti.*

14. This is made even clearer by Cakrapāṇidatta's commentary on *Suśruta.*, Sū 24.7 (Sū 24.5 in *Suśruta*[1].). According to him, *upasarga-* refers to diseases which are sudden/accidental (*ākasmika-*), and arise in persons afflicted (*upasṛṣṭa-*, from *upa*$\sqrt{}$*sṛj*) by attacks etc. (*abhighātādi-*) [and?] by angry gods etc., as an explanation of which he quotes *Suśruta.*, Ni 5.34.[25] But Ni 5.33 f with its mention of *aupasargika-* (see §4) was the starting point of our discussion, seemingly being a straightforward description of diseases being transmitted by the sort of "natural" contagion we as a rule mean when using the expression *contagion*. Cakrapāṇidatta goes on to quote, not directly with regard to *upasarga-*, but in the larger context of diseases originating through divine power, *Caraka.*, Ci 9.18, which tells us that gods etc., not spoiling/injuring (*adūṣayat-*) the body of a man, invisibly and speedily enter this through the power of their own properties, like a reflection the mirror or sunlight the suncrystal (*sūryakānta-*). This is then connected with the theory of retribution for former deeds. To underscore this, *Caraka.*, Vi 3.22 and 23 are quoted, which speak of supernatural retribution for *adharma-*.[26] The twofold differentiation of diseases according to whether they are caused by lightning or thunder, or by *piśāca-*s etc., is connected by him with *upasarga-* only; under the affliction through *piśāca-*s and the like he wishes to subsume the afflictions described as part of the devastation of countries (*janapadoddhvaṃsana-*),[27] which is quite clearly a reference to *Caraka.*, Vi 3, a chapter in which the devastation of countries, not only, but also through epidemics, is described, the main cause being given as non-adherence to *dharma-*, namely *adharma-* (thus also in the passages already quoted), i.e., what we from our modern point of view tend to call immorality or unethical behaviour.[28] Finally, Cakrapāṇidatta explains diseases arising due to *saṃsarga-* as arising due to contact/connection/association (*saṃsarga-*) with persons with *aupasargika-* diseases. Explaining this further, he says that those which arise due to con-

---

[25] *upasargā ity ākasmikarogāḥ. te hi kruddhadevādyabhighātādyupasṛṣṭasya bhavantīty upasargā ucyante. yad uktam "aupasargikarogāś ca saṅkrāmanti narān naram" iti.*

[26] *abhicārābhiśāpābhiṣaṅgajā iti. abhicāraḥ kṛtyā. abhiśāpo guruvṛddhasiddhācāryādibhir abhiśapanam. abhiṣaṅgo devādīnāṃ viparyayeṇānupraveśaḥ. yad uktaṃ carake "devādayaḥ svair hi guṇaprabhāvair adūṣayantaḥ puruṣasya deham viśanty adṛśyās tarasā yathaiva cchāyātapau darpaṇasūryakāntau" iti. ete 'bhicārādayaḥ prāktanāśubhakarmapākavaśād eva puruṣam upaghnanti. yad uktaṃ carake "rakṣogaṇādibhir vā vividhair bhūtasaṅghais tam adharmam anyad vāpy apacārāntaram upalabhyābhihanyante". "tathābhiśāpaprabhavasyāpy adharma eva hetur" ityādi. tena daivaṃ prāktanaṃ karmābhivartata ity adhidaivam.*

[27] *atha piśācādikṛtena janapadoddhvaṃsanabhavāś cāntarbhāvanīyāḥ.*

[28] Whether we would be right in doing so will be discussed below.

tact/connection/association (*saṃsarga-*) with *kuṣṭha-*[29] etc. originate due to the power of the morbific entities because they arise due to the morbific entities of the body; those which arise due to contact/connection/association (*saṃsarga-*) with *aupasargika-* diseases, however, originate in *adharma-*.[30]

15. All of this is admittedly more than a little confusing, but the general drift of the material sifted does allow the deduction that what we have so far regarded as contagion is in fact somewhat removed from our modern understanding of the term. There seems to be some component in all this which from our modern point of view we would label "supernatural". That this impression is justified is shown by other passages in the texts examined, passages not systematically searched for, but chosen at random, which means that a systematic search will most probably turn up many more examples.

16. In *Aṣṭāṅgasaṃgraha*, Ut 49(page 417b) the plant *somarājī-*[31] is said to keep away poison, evil spirits (*bhūta-*), *upasarga-* and *pāpman-* when kept in the house. Now *pāpman-* is "badness",[32] and at least according to later Vedic texts a mite, to our eyes, supernatural.[33] The position of *upasarga-* between this and evil spirits does make it seem as if it too were something we would analyse as supernatural. Against this one could for instance point to *Aṣṭāṅgasaṃgraha*, Sū 3(22a), where one is warned not to frequent a site which is (in this order) condemned by the texts pertaining to the knowledge of sites,[34] full of diseases, without physicians, without a leader, with a majority of people given to *adharma-* (i.e., what we today would call morally or ethically lacking), which is *upasṛṣṭa-*, and a mountain.[35] Now *upasṛṣṭa-* is the past participle of *upa*$\sqrt{}$*sṛj*; in a context such as this its most neutral translation is probably "adhered to", which could mean "afflicted", but need not, as it may have other shades of meaning. The commentator Indu explains it as "with *upasarga-*s,

---

[29] Cf. note 4.

[30] *atra saṃsargajā aupasargikarogisaṃsargajātāḥ. ye tu kuṣṭhādisaṃsargajās te śārīradoṣajatayā doṣabalapravṛttā eva. aupasargikarogasaṃsargajās tv adharmabhūtā evety ādhidaivike 'ntarbhavanti.* It is noteworthy that Cakrapāṇidatta first speaks of contact with persons having certain diseases, and then of contact with diseases themselves. Or is *aupasargikarogisaṃsargajātāḥ* actually a mistake for *aupasargikarogasaṃsargajātāḥ*?

[31] Here alluded to by the epithet *rekhā cāndramasī.*

[32] See *pāpa-* in §§6 f.

[33] See on this note 11.

[34] That is, *vāstuśāstra-*, usually translated as "architecture", though it does not pertain only to buildings.

[35] *naikāham apy adhivased vāstu tacchāstragarhitam*
na deśaṃ vyādhibahulaṃ nāvaidyaṃ nāpy anāyakam
nādharmijanabhūyiṣṭhaṃ nopasṛṣṭaṃ na parvatam.

[i.e.] together with deadly epidemics etc.".[36] Be that as it may, *upasṛṣṭa-*, even though it comes right after *adharma-*, could be taken to be something in our eyes quite "natural", especially since it comes right before the mention of a mountain. This could mean that our understanding of *Aṣṭāṅgasaṃgraha*, Ut 49(417b) too is faulty. On the other hand, we must also ask why a mountain is to be avoided; after all, is not mountain air good for health? The answer seems to me to lie in the fact that in most cultures[37] around the earth, India being no exception, mountains are considered to be the abode of supernatural beings, and as such both holy and dangerous. Though we can ultimately only speculate on the *Aṣṭāṅgasaṃgraha* passage quoted, this would seem to be a good reason for it to mention a mountain as a place to avoid, from which it would follow that *upasṛṣṭa-* too may very well refer to something to us supernatural.

17. The connection between *upasṛṣṭa-* and something supernatural is quite pronounced in *Suśruta.*, Sū 1.8,4, where the purpose of *bhūtavidyā-* "the knowledge of evil spirits"[38] is explained as the pacification (*upaśama-*) by various means of the *graha-*s of those whose intellect (*cetas-*) is *upasṛṣṭa-* by gods and various other good and bad superhuman beings, manes, flesh-eating demons (*piśāca-*), serpent-beings (*nāga-*), *graha-*s, etc. The word *graha-* is quite common in the meaning "planet", but in medical texts it oftener denotes a class of non-human beings, mostly, but not only, malevolent, that are responsible for various sorts of disorders, in the case of adults usually mental, but in the case of children mostly of various bodily sorts. There are several cases in *Suśruta.* of *graha-* being combined with a form of *upa*√*sṛj* to denote someone afflicted by a disorder due to *graha-*s; Śā 10.46 and 50 mention the *upasarga-* by or through *graha-*s (*grahopasarga-*) as something to guard against, whereas Śā 10.51, Ut 28.3 and Ut 37.21 speak of persons who are *upasṛṣṭa-* by or through *graha-*s (*grahopasṛṣṭa-*). These latter occurrences make it improbable that *grahopasarga-* in *Suśruta.* is a copulative compound, even though in

[36] *upasṛṣṭaṃ sopasargaṃ* (variant: *sopasṛṣṭam* "with [what is] *upasṛṣṭa-*", which seems meaningless) *mārakādinā.*

[37] I hope I will be excused for using a term here of which it has recently been said: "So it seems that there are now quite a number of anthropologists who, when they hear the word 'culture', will reach for their guns" (98 of Ulf Hannerz, "When Culture is Everywhere: Reflections on a Favorite Concept," *Ethnos* 58 ⟨1993⟩: 95–111). Even though I admit to being at a loss how exactly to define the term I am using here, I am confident that my readers will nevertheless not have difficulties in understanding me.

[38] Cf. note 19.

Aṣṭāṅgasaṃgraha, Ut 49(429a) *graha-* and *upasarga-* are clearly parallel members of a copulative compound, separated by *maraka-* "deadly epidemic".

18. Now of course the fact that *upa√sṛj* and its derivatives can be used in contexts in which forces we would tend to label as supernatural are at work does not mean that when used in the context of transmission of diseases they must have such supernatural connections too. But at least we are now able to say that the usage of the words in connection with what is to us supernatural has been shown not to be impossible, so that the supernatural connections native commentators have made in this context (cf. §§6 f and §§11 ff.) are not ruled out by the use of *upa√sṛj* or its derivatives—and may indeed even be held to be substantiated by our discussion above.

19. In §14 we have seen a native commentator connecting the transmission of diseases with what we would call moral or ethical considerations (see also §16). In this context it is very interesting to find Gayadāsa in his commentary on *Suśruta.*, Ni 5.33 f, already discussed in §§4 ff., making the very same connection. Commenting on the diseases listed as being transmitted by various sorts of contact, he says that these diseases (explained by him as "pox etc.") which *Suśruta.* calls *aupasargika-*, arise due to general[39] *adharma-* (*sāmānyādharmapravṛtta-*). To explain the verb used to describe the transmission, namely *saṅkrāmanti*, he uses the verb *āviśanti*, which we have already met in §6. Explaining how this happens, he says that through connection/intercourse[40] (*prasaṅga-*) with those indulging in *pāpa-* (*pāpakṛt-*), *pāpa-* passes on/over/through (*saṅkramati*); *pāpa-* has already been explained in §§6 f (cf. also *pāpman-* in §16). In this context he then quotes *Caraka.*, Sū 1.130, which says:

> "Even through conversing with him a man falls into Hell."[41]

From this it is clear that to Gayadāsa those indulging in something which we from our modern point of view would call immoral or unethical manifest

[39] I am unsure whether this is the correct translation for *sāmānya-* in the given context; in any case, I do not know what exactly is meant.

[40] Cf. note 6.

[41] *naro narakapātī syāt tasya sambhāṣaṇād api.* The whole portion of the commentary paraphrased above runs: *aupasargikā rogāḥ sāmānyādharmapravṛttā masūrādayaḥ. saṅkrāmanti narān naram āviśanti. tad eva katham. pāpakṛtāṃ prasaṅgena pāpaṃ saṅkramati. tad uktaṃ carake*
"naro narakapātī syāt tasya sambhāṣanād api"
iti. rogaprabhāvād ity anye. The last sentence translates as: "Others [say]: 'Due to the power/faculty of (or: as a consequence of/through) (*prabhāvāt*) the disease'." On this see note 66.

some sort of disease, and that through contact with these persons something is passed on to others, to describe which the same term is used as for what is indulged in.

20. What makes the whole even more intriguing is the fact that the passage from *Caraka.* which Gayadāsa quotes is actually part of quite another context, for *Caraka.*, Sū 1.129 f say:

> "The physician who, without knowing the [correct] treatment, holding himself to be knowledgeable, offers [treatment] to the suffering, bedridden, trusting patient: even through conversing with him (the physician), the *pāpa-* one by whom *dharma-* has been forsaken, who is death itself (literally: who has become death),[42] whose disposition of mind is bad, a man falls into Hell."[43]

For us there seems to be no connection between a bad physician of this sort and the transmission of disease. Now one could say that Gayadāsa has simply selected part of this passage out of context, and applied it to what he is commenting upon. On the other hand, it is hard to believe that he would be oblivious to the fact that the medical specialists for whom his commentary is ultimately meant would surely be aware of the context from which he had taken his quotation. After all, they too would most probably have been familiar with the same text of *Caraka.* as Gayadāsa. So it does seem very probable—though of course we cannot prove this beyond the shadow of a doubt—that Gayadāsa actually means to make a connection between the passage from *Caraka.* and the passage from *Suśruta.* he is commenting upon. In other words, whatever evil or the like overcomes the bad physician through his condemnable act is to Gayadāsa of the same category as that which has overcome those suffering from certain diseases because of something they have done, and the transference of whatever it is that affects these latter through contact with them is basically of the same sort as the misfortune that overtakes one having contact with the bad physician. Interesting is also the fact that we cannot be sure that what overcomes the bad physician and can be transferred to others is the

---

[42]Variant: "the *pāpa-* messenger of death, by whom *dharma-* has been forsaken".

[43] *duḥkhitāya śayānāya śraddadhānāya rogiṇe*
yo bheṣajam avijñāya prājñamānī prayacchati
tyaktadharmasya pāpasya mṛtyubhūtasya durmateḥ
naro narakapātī syāt tasya sambhāṣaṇād api.
The variant has *mṛtyudūtasya* for *mṛtyubhūtasya.*

same as what we would call diseases or the like; for all we know it may be something else that has adverse effects as diseases have, especially since one can hardly assume that the bad physician is always ill.

21. This seeming sameness of the effects of what in our eyes are actions or the like belonging to quite different spheres, namely the spheres of morality or ethics and natural causes, brings to mind the devastation of countries (which includes epidemics) through *adharma-* drawn attention to in §14. We find this same equivalence in *Suśruta.*, Sū 6.19 too. After in the foregoing passages detailing the adverse effects, including epidemics (*maraka-*), of certain environmental conditions, the text lists other environmental causes for the same effects, heading this list with sorcery, curses, anger of demons and *adharma-*, which, it says, devastate countries.

22. If however natural and what in our eyes would be moral or ethical factors may bring about the same or similar adverse results, which may even be transmitted, then it stands to reason that the same sort of danger emanates from those with what to us would be moral or ethical faults as from those with what to us are infectious diseases. And it also stands to reason that those refusing to acknowledge the correctness of and uphold the prevailing notions of what we would today term morals or ethics are potentially especially dangerous, since their disbelief must lead them to actions or the like which are not in keeping with these prevailing notions. Is it for this reason that *Suśruta.*, Sū 34.21 f describes the ideal patient as one who is, amongst other things, an *āstika-*, i.e., one who believes in the existence of the supra-human, an after-life and all that is associated with these concepts? And is it for the same reason that the chief among those patients to be avoided and not to be treated, serving as the example *par excellence* for this type of patient, is according to *Caraka.*, Sū 25.40 and *Aṣṭāṅgasaṃgraha*, Sū 13(111b) the *nāstika-*, the one who negates the beliefs of the *āstika-*?

23. There is yet another point to consider. In §§19 f we mentioned a passage stating that even conversing with certain persons might lead to harmful effects. We could hold that this is not meant literally, but is to be understood as saying that even the slightest contact may be harmful. But what if the statement is to be taken literally, namely that conversing, not necessarily with any sort of actual contact (even via breath) having taken place, is harmful? This question has to be asked because of a passage quoted by the *Kairalī* commentary on *Aṣṭāṅgahṛdaya.*, Ut 31.8 (see *Aṣṭāṅgahṛdaya.*[2]) and Indu in his commentary on *Aṣṭāṅgasaṃgraha*, Ut 36(269a) and attributed to the ancient authority Urabhra. This says:

> "Through seeing, touching [and] giving [of gifts or the like], diseases of the skin and eyes, epilepsy (*apasmāra-*), kingly consumption (*rājayakṣman-*)[44] and pustules (*masūrikā-*) pass on/over/through (*saṅkrāmanti*) from man to man."[45]

There can be no doubt that this verse attributed to Urabhra actually does describe a transference of disease by a process, namely seeing, that we would not associate with such transference. It is also interesting to note that the last part of this passage is identical to the last part of *Suśruta.*, Ni 5.33 f translated in §4.

24. Let us now recapitulate what we have deduced from the discussion so far. There seems to be evidence to presume that the differentiation between heredity and contagion we make with regard to transference of diseases might not have been made in the Indian medical texts discussed here. We also found that the transference affected not only diseases and the like which arise through what to us are natural causes, but also those which arise through what to us are supernatural causes; one passage even says that all or almost all diseases are transferable (see §2). Moreover, we cannot be sure that it is only diseases that are so transferred; this possibility presents itself especially in connection with the adverse effects of what we would call moral or ethical wrong-doing (cf. §20). And finally, we have seen that the transference may also take place by means of actions not involving any sort of contact as we today understand it, e.g., by speaking with or looking at certain persons.

25. Is there any way in which we can explain all this? I think that there is. The various notions seemingly connected with transference of diseases etc. fit what I have elsewhere called the "magical mode of looking at the world". Actually, this is a rather clumsy attempt to translate the German *magisches Weltbild* or *magische Weltanschauung*, especially because "magical" in English has connotations different from the German *magisch*; I can, however, think of no other equivalent, unless one prefers the commonly used "magico-religious" in the place of "magical", which however leads right into the midst of the well-known and as yet unresolved controversy on the relationship between magic and religion,[46] a controversy which ultimately might not even be relevant in the ancient Indian context.

---

[44] On this disease see especially Meulenbeld (see note 1), 628 f.

[45] *tvagakṣirogāpasmārarājayakṣmamasūrikāḥ*
darśanāt sparśanād dānāt saṅkrāmanti narān naram.

[46] See on this problem also 13[5] of Rahul Peter Das, "Heilsvorstellungen in der altindischen ('hinduistischen') Medizin," in *Religionen und medizinische Ethik.* Mit Beiträgen von Rahul

26. The *magische*[47] *Weltbild* (if I be allowed the use of the German expression here) in its Indian form is known best from later Vedic literature, particularly the class of texts called the Brāhmaṇas. But we also have a lot of evidence for its existence in later times, and this includes the medical literature we are here concerned with. The characteristics of this *magische Weltbild* have been set forth and discussed elsewhere,[48] so that it suffices to give a very brief overview here. In short, the "magical mode of looking at the world" seems characterized by a non-differentiation between living and non-living, concrete and abstract, corporeal and non-corporeal. The world consists of "powers" (also called "mights", "substances", "entities" or something similar) in various states or forms, which are however not immutable; such powers can take control of each other and manifest themselves, wholly or in part, through what has been taken control of. Taking control can happen through voluntary action of the power or through its being made to act by others; the path of taking control may be actual physical contact either directly (to which hereditary affiliation also belongs) or indirectly (e.g., through breath, the use of common implements etc.), but, since thoughts, words and deeds are not basically different, also by other means. The powers are also interconnected in a system of mutual balance or order, so that any action (which includes thoughts, words and the like), be it ever so small, must create a disturbance and cause a reaction; since this applies to each and every action, there is obviously no separation between the secular and the sacral.[49] It is however possible

Peter Das, Mirko Frýba, Robert Jütte, Adel Theodor Khoury, Ina Rösing Diederich, Bausteine zur Philosophie 7 (Ulm: Humboldt-Studienzentrum, Universität Ulm, 1993): 11–40.

[47] I am treating the English article like the German article and therefore changing the declension of the German adjective accordingly.

[48] See Rahul Peter Das, "[Review of:] G. U. Thite. Medicine. Its Magico-Religious Aspects according to the Vedic and Later Literature. Poona 1982," *Indo-Iranian Journal* 27 (1984): 232–44, with further bibliographic references, as well as 201 ff. of *Idem*, "[Review of:] Stanley Jeyaraja Tambiah. Magic, science, religion and the scope of rationality. Cambridge etc. 1990," *Journal of the European Āyurvedic Society* 2 (1992): 200–4.

[49] A well-known example is found in the tale of King Nala in the *Mahābhārata*. Kali, the worst and losing throw in dicing, tries in vain for twelve years to gain possession of Nala. Finally he sees his chance when Nala forgets to wash his feet before performing the ritual acts at the juncture of two divisions of the day; he enters Nala at once, upon which Nala plays at dice and loses everything, including his kingdom. The incident of Kali is narrated in 3.56.2 ff. of the critical edition of the *Mahābhārata*; note that the verb forms used to describe how Kali enters Nala are *āviśat* and *samāviśya*, from *(sam)-ā√viś*, which bring to mind another form of *ā√viś*, namely *āviśanti*, in §6 and §19 above. I may also add that the continuation of the story of Nala makes it clear that only a part of Kali has entered Nala, which is in keeping with what

to take preventive measures to counteract the results of certain actions, and for this background knowledge of the various powers and what they can do is the most efficient means.

27. Of course what we regard as diseases are in this mode of looking at the world powers too, which manifest themselves in humans. But such diseases are not the only means of manifestation, other manifestations (which may even include things such as ugliness, foul-mouthedness and so on) being equally possible. In this regard it must also be emphasized that the power and what we have called its manifestation are not something different, but one and the same, since the manifestation is in fact the power itself, though it may not be the whole power. Actually, our categories of thought and speech at times make it very difficult to express this adequately, and this is also the case as regards our differentiation of the abstract and the concrete, which may even force us to look for the concretization of something abstract or the abstraction of something concrete when in fact no such differentiation exists. Similarly, we would probably be forced to differentiate between an action someone does due to being overwhelmed by a power, and this power itself, whereas actually the action is not different from, for instance, some physical characteristic, and but a manifestation of the power and thus ultimately this power too.

28. Since the notions of the later Vedic texts certainly did not appear out of thin air, and since similar notions are found all over the world, it stands to reason that they must have been present in earlier Vedic times too. There is however a controversy on how extensive these notions were in earlier times, but this is basically irrelevant in our context,[50] since we are here concerned primarily with post-Vedic times. Now as regards these latter, it cannot of course be claimed that "magical" notions are the only ones present, or even that they are predominant, but that they are present to at least some degree even in modern Indian society is a commonplace, and hardly surprising

---

has just been said above on the manifestation of powers.

[50] I would however like to draw attention to the remarks in Das, "Heilsvorstellungen in der altindischen ('hinduistischen') Medizin," 13 f. With regard to the question of whether the gods in the Vedic Saṃhitās too may be powers, I must also draw attention to G. E. Dunkel ("Vater Himmels Gattin," *Die Sprache* 34 ⟨1988–90⟩: 1–26, and 35 ⟨1991–3⟩: 1), who explains some of them (Varuṇa, Parjanya, Indra) naturalistically as originally epithets of a god "Father Heaven"; unfortunately, the remarks on this subject are apodictic and not accompanied by any in-depth study of the gods remarked upon, so that the last word on this subject has clearly not been spoken yet.

given the fact that modern Western societies too harbour remnants of such notions.[51]

29. Coming now to the field of Indian medicine, it is highly interesting to note that Emmerick[52] analyses the terms used to describe diseases in Indo-Iranian and comes to the conclusion that they nearly all are etymologically connected with the concept of "seizing" or the like, thus being clearly connected to the overwhelming by some adverse power of the sort described above. We too have in §17 already come across a word having a similar origin, namely *graha-*, whose basic meaning is "seizer".[53] Now there is no denying the fact that in the medical texts we are concerned with *graha-*, like other "disease" words derived from the concept of "seizing", has mostly been replaced by other words for "disease" not having similar origins,[54] but we have seen above that this has by no means led to its being discarded; on the contrary, we even found that it plays a role in the context of transmission of diseases. It may also be noted that in *Madanamahārṇava* 40, where the actions of and measures against various *graha-*s are described, we find not only *graha-*s like those in the other medical works discussed here mentioned, but also a "fever *graha-*" (*jvaragraha-*),[55] which is said to seize (*gṛhṇāti*, from the same verbal root as *graha-*) especially those guilty of what we would call moral offences, *adharma-* being specifically mentioned in this connection (444 f).

---

[51] On the notion of everything without exception being living in later Indian philosophical speculation see now especially Walter Slaje, "Merkmale des Lebendigen: Zu einer naturphilosophisch begründeten Biologie in Bhāskarakaṇṭhas *Cittānubodhaśāstra,* " *Journal of the European Āyurvedic Society* 3 (1993): 250–81.

[52] Ronald E. Emmerick, "Indo-Iranian Concepts of Disease and Cure," *Journal of the European Āyurvedic Society* 3 (1993): 72–93; see 84 ff.

[53] Since this usage of the word in medical contexts is not already Indo-Iranian, Emmerick did not examine it.

[54] Whether *graha-* in combination with various body parts to denote an affliction of that part (e.g., *hṛdgraha-* with *hṛd-* "heart", *galagraha-* with *gala-* "throat") is derived from a usage of *graha-* like that detailed above, or whether *graha-* here actually has some other meaning, has to my knowledge not been examined yet.

[55] I have also found the expression *jvaragraha-* in *Siddhasāra* 5.117, but here it is unclear whether we indeed have "fever *graha-*" or simply a copulative compound "fever and *graha-*s". cf. also *Harivaṃśa* (edition used: *The Harivaṁśa being the Khila or Supplement to the Mahābhārata. Volume II (Appendices),* ed. Parashuram Lakshman Vaidya ⟨Poona: Bhandarkar Oriental Research Institute, 1971⟩), Appendix I, no.24, lines 113–57, where various entities are called upon for protection; here *jvara-*s are mentioned in line 114 and *graha-*s in line 135, as well as various individual *graha-*s later on, but since there are text-critical problems connected with the passage, the relationship between *jvara-*s and *graha-*s is unclear.

30. This brings up once again the matter of what we today would call the moral or ethical component drawn attention to several times in our discussion above, and which is also found in discussions on the causes of disease in non-medical works.[56] In the context of "magical" thought such English terminology does not, however, make sense, and it thus is no surprise that in our discussion of the medical texts above we came across many examples of what to us would belong to different categories (natural, supernatural, moral/ethical) not being differentiated, in the same way as diseases and other things adverse to humans seem not to have been clearly differentiated.[57] In this connection I would like to draw particular attention to the references to *pāpa-* and *pāpman-* above, particularly in §19. The reason I am singling out these expressions is that one of the very few known terms for individual diseases going back to Indo-Iranian times is *pāmán-* (this is the Indian form of the word), which denotes some sort of skin disease;[58] this word could, however, be etymologically connected with *pāpa-* and *pāpman-*. The connection, also found in the passage translated in §6, of the latter with another skin disease, namely *kuṣṭha-*, should also be noted in this connection; in *Suśruta.*, Ni 5.30 too, *kuṣṭha-* is called a *pāpa-* disease, which appears in those who do actions such as killing Brahmins, women and good people, taking for themselves what rightfully belongs to others, etc. Even today one finds the belief that *kuṣṭha-* (whose modern linguistic descendants have mostly taken on the more specialized meaning of "leprosy") arises due to what we would call immoral or unethical deeds to be widespread in India.[59]

31. Now two expressions which we today tend to associate with moral and ethical concepts have cropped up several times in our discussion so far,

---

[56] See on this latter point e.g., Wezler (see note 17), 144 ff., where there are also further references, as well as 118 ff. of Lallanji Gopal, "Devala and Ayurveda," in *Studies in Orientology. Essays in memory of Prof. A. L. Basham*, ed. S. K. Maity, Upendra Thakur and A. K. Narain (Agra: Y. K. Publishers, 1988), 113–23.

[57] In this context it is worthy of note that hunger and thirst, in Indo-Iranian times probably thought to be the manifestations of harmful powers (see Emmerick, "Indo-Iranian Concepts of Disease and Cure", 91), are even in the medical texts examined here classified on a par with diseases, something quite against our mode of thinking. (On the subject of hunger and thirst being classified as diseases attention may also be drawn to Reinhold F. G. Müller, "A szomjúság (és az éhség) indiai orvosok értékelésében," and "Durst (und Hunger), bewertet durch indische Ärzte," *Communicationes ex Bibliotheca Historiae Medicae Hungarica* 21/22 ⟨1961⟩: 30–40 and 41–53).

[58] See also Emmerick, ibid., 90.

[59] Of course this belief was or is not confined to India, as several other contributions to this volume too show.

namely the expression *dharma-* and its opposite, *adharma-*. But what exactly is *dharma-*? It is a commonplace to Indologists that it is a system (of unclear contours) of rules which govern practically every aspect of life, rules which are just there and have not been formulated by any known individuals, though they may be codified by them.[60] Yet at the same time we have examples galore which seem to say that *dharma-* is also something substantial. Not only that, it seems at times also to be something which can be done. If we now compare this with what has been said above on powers (especially §§26 f), we find that the characteristics of *dharma-* seem to be in striking agreement with those of powers, whilst at the same time the fact that *dharma-* regulates all one does, and that its infringement even in matters to us moderns quite unimportant may have grave results, reminds us of the notions of mutual interconnectedness of all powers, due to which anything one does is bound to have repercussions of some, but not necessarily of the same, sort. These characteristics of *dharma-* have of course also been seen by others, the to my knowledge best example for this being the explanation of *dharma-* attempted by Paul Hacker on 506 of his collected works,[61] which I am here translating from the original German:[62]

> "The *dharma-* is, rather, a concrete, positive-salutary[63] *behavioural model* that somehow exists even before being carried out and awaits realisation, or a collection of such models. Dharma *being carried out* is then that act corresponding to this model, Adharma that contrary to it. Finally, the Dharma-substance,

[60] Such codices are however anything but uniform, not only because they contain only certain selected rules, but also because such rules in general are not static, nor necessarily the same for all. On this aspect of *dharma-* attention may now also be drawn to Ludo Rocher, "Law Books in an Oral Culture: The Indian *Dharmaśāstras*," *Proceedings of the American Philosophical Society Held at Philadelphia for Promoting Useful Knowledge* 137 (1993): 254–67 (particularly 266 f).

[61] Paul Hacker, *Kleine Schriften*, ed. Lambert Schmithausen, Glasenapp-Stiftung 15 (Wiesbaden: Franz Steiner Verlag, 1978).

[62] "Der Dharma ist vielmehr ein konkretes, positiv-heilswertiges *Verhaltensmodell*, das schon vor dem Vollzug irgendwie existiert und auf Realisierung wartet, bzw. eine Sammlung solcher Modelle. Dharma *im Vollzug* ist dann das diesem Modell entsprechende, Adharma das ihm widersprechende Handeln. Schließlich existiert die Dharmasubstanz aber auch noch *nach dem Vollzug* als das realisierte Verhaltensmodell. Es ist dann so etwas wie ein zu einem übersinnlichen Wirkstoff geronnenes Tun, die Substanz der getanen Tat."

[63] I am not sure whether this is the correct translation of *positiv-heilswertig*.

however, also exists *after being carried out* as the realised behavioural model. It is then something like an action congealed to supersensory effective matter, the substance of the done deed."

32. An examination of whether this explanation of *dharma-* (and *adharma-*) is fitting or not cannot be attempted here. What is relevant in our context is that this explanation also expresses what must strike one after our discussion of the medical material above, and this is all the more so when we consider that the transference of diseases we are here concerned with finds a parallel in what is among scholars usually termed the "transference of merit and demerit", which is quite clearly linked with the concepts of *dharma-* and *adharma-*.[64] In the light of the non-differentiation of diseases and other adverse things referred to in §30, such parallels are clearly very intriguing; they are yet another piece of evidence allowing us to arrive at not only a description of what "contagion" in the Indian medical context actually is, but also an explanation of why its mention in Indian medical texts is not very frequent.

33. It seems that what we term "contagion" is in the ancient Indian context actually part of a complex of notions ultimately going back to the "magical mode of looking at the world". Diseases are only one of the various means by which the powers that make up the world may manifest themselves in humans after they have overpowered or penetrated them. The modes of overpowering or penetration are various, and include physical contact either directly or indirectly, but also other means of what obviously was taken to be contact too, such as looking or hearing,[65] as well as acts (leading to a reaction on the part of the power) which we would rather classify as of a moral or ethical nature. Since all this is to be seen in the context of the interconnectedness of everything, it is obvious that there is actually no need for a special treatment of the matter with regard to medicine or diseases, since the rules governing life generally (i.e., *dharma-*) are applicable in such contexts as well. This would explain why so little of relevance particularly to the matter concerning us here is to be found in medical texts. Moreover, since everything, be it good or bad, is but a manifestation of some power and thus ultimately this power (cf. §27), there is theoretically no limit to what can be transmitted; the statement in §2

[64] On this latter subject see now especially Albrecht Wezler, "The Warrior Taking to Flight in Fear. Some Remarks on Manu 7.94 and 95. (Beiträge zur Kenntnis der indischen Kultur- und Religionsgeschichte III)," *Indologica Taurinensia* 14 (1987–8): 391–432, particularly 421 ff.

[65] These same means can also be used to drive away a power. One need only think of the effects of substances such as Ganges water or holy basil in this context; but equal effects can also be achieved by the seeing, hearing etc. of "auspicious" things.

that all or almost all diseases pass from one person to another is quite consistent with this belief, though it does not preclude that, since not all powers are equally mighty, some diseases may be transmitted more than others.

34. Of course it would be quite naïve to maintain that notions such as those set forth here are all that we have to consider in our study of Indian medical texts or society in general,[66] but it has to be admitted that they do serve well in explaining much of the material that we have analysed in the course of our small study.[67] It also stands to reason that in a situation of constant mutual interconnectedness the best way to avoid not only disease, but anything unpleasant, is to constantly guard against doing something which would bring about disharmony amongst the various mutually balanced powers, with potentially harmful results. In this context the so-called "ritual purity", so often mentioned in connection with India,[68] makes eminent sense, though clearly the adjective "ritual" is, in the light of what we have seen so far, quite out of place here. And since there is, contrary to our modern way of thinking, basically no difference between the results of thoughts, words and deeds in this regard, the Indian emphasis on both external and internal purity that has struck scholars again and again is not at all surprising.

35. Now our findings above are based only on a handful of Indian medical texts, so that they remain in need of verification through studies of other medical texts, as well as of medical matter found in texts not primarily of a

---

[66]This seems also to be hinted at by the last sentence of Gayadāsa's commentary quoted in note 41, which one could understand as being criticism against the notion of some sort of might or the like being involved here.

[67]It must also be emphasized that several of these notions seem to have close parallels in other cultures of the earth, as borne witness to not only by the other contributions to this volume of which this essay is a part, but also the other contributions of the volume containing Das, "Heilsvorstellungen in der altindischen ('hinduistischen') Medizin". In this context we may recollect what Bernfried Schlerath wrote in another context ("Zu den Merseburger Zaubersprüchen," *II. Fachtagung für Indogermanische und Allgemeine Sprachwissenschaft Innsbruck, 10.–15. Oktober 1961. Vorträge und Veranstaltungen*, Innsbrucker Beiträge zur Kulturwissenschaft, Sonderheft 15 ⟨Innsbruck: Sprachwissenschaftliches Institut der Leopold-Franzens-Universität Innsbruck, 1962⟩, 139–43): "Die Völkerkunde hat uns mit einer unübersehbaren Fülle von Material bekannt gemacht, das zwar von einer faszinierenden Buntheit ist, das uns aber an den verschiedensten Enden der Welt immer wieder die erstaunlichsten Parallelen zeigt. Mir ist es noch nicht begegnet, daß ein Völkerkundler, dem ich eine Einzelheit aus der Vorstellungswelt der Idg. [= Indogermanistik] vortrug, nicht sofort eine Reihe von engen Parallelen aus naturvölkischem Bereich zur Hand hatte" (140).

[68]And often leading to remarks which we may, if we be allowed to call a spade a spade, bluntly label as nonsense, such as the notion, seemingly quite popular among some North American scholars, that Indian "ritual purity" is the outcome of a male castration complex!

medical nature,[69] though I personally doubt that such further studies will lead to any major revision of our findings. In any case, the evidence we have found for ancient notions going back to the Vedic age still being very influential in later texts should make those scholars who hold that there is a clear break between Vedic and later medicine reconsider their position.[70]

ABBREVIATIONS

Aṣṭāṅgahṛdaya. *Aṣṭāṅgahṛdayam (The Core of Octopartite Āyurveda) composed by Vāgbhaṭa With the Commentaries (Sarvāṅgasundarā) of Aruṇadatta and (Āyurvedarasāyana) of Hemādri,* collated by Aṇṇā Moreśwara Kuṇṭe and Kṛṣṇa Rāmchandra Śāstrī Navare, ed. Hariśāstrī Parāḍakara Vaidya, Jaikrishnadas Ayurveda Series 52 (Varanasi: Chaukhambha Orientalia, ^{7}1982).

Aṣṭāṅgahṛdaya.^{1} *Aṣṭāṅgarḍaya ⟨sic⟩ of Vāhaṭa With the Commentary Hṛdayabodhikā of Śrīdāsapaṇḍita. Part III (Śārīrasthāna and Nidānasthāna),* ed. K. Raghavan Pillai, Trivandrum Sanskrit Series 201 (Trivandrum: University of Kerala, 1962).

Aṣṭāṅgahṛdaya.^{2} *ŚrīmadVāhaṭaviracitaṃ Aṣṭāṃgahṛdayaṃ—uttarasthānam. Kairalīvyākhyayā samullasitam,* ed. Vayaskarāgāranivāsin Nārāyaṇaśarmātmaaja Śaṃkaraśarman and Ceppāṭ Ke. Acyutavārya, Vaidyasārathigrantha-āvali 1 (Koṭṭayam: Vaidyasārathimudraṇālaya, 1942).

Aṣṭāṅgasaṃgraha *Aṣṭāṅgasaṅgrahaḥ. Induvyākhyāsahitaḥ,* ed. Ṭi. Rudrapāraśava (Trichur: The Mangalodayam Press, 1913–26) (3 volumes).

Caraka. *The Charakasaṃhitā by Agniveśa Revised by Charaka and Dṛidhabala ⟨sic⟩ With the Āyurveda-Dīpikā Commentary of Chakrapāṇidatta,* ed. Jādavaji Trikamji Āchārya, reprinted, The Kashi Sanskrit Series 228 (Varanasi: Chaukhambha Sanskrit Sansthan, 1984).

---

[69] Some relevant material from the latter is found on 52 f of P. V. Sharma, *Indian Medicine in the Classical Age,* The Chowkhamba Sanskrit Studies 85 (Varanasi: Chowkhamba Sanskrit Series Office, 1972).

[70] "Scientific" or "rational" later Indian medicine is often sharply contrasted with "magico-religious" or "irrational" Vedic medicine by scholars. On this problem with regard to Indian medicine see e.g., the discussion on 162 ff. of Rahul Peter Das, "Indische Medizin und Spiritualität," *Journal of the European Āyurvedic Society* 2 (1992): 158–87. It should also be noted that many of the difficulties encountered in discussing this problem centre on the haziness of the term "rational", which is nevertheless more often than not used as if it were perfectly clear to all concerned what is meant; cf. in this regard also Jack Goody, "East and West: Rationality in Review," *Ethnos* 58 (1993): 6–36 (esp. 31 ff.), though his linkage of what he calls "rationality or logic" (e.g., on page 10) with written cultures, in which context he also cites the grammar of Sanskrit by Pāṇini, will surely be challenged by those who hold that ancient Indian culture was basically oral, but nevertheless brought forth such scholarly monuments as Pāṇini's grammar, the linkage of such intellectual feats with writing being but a projection of the modern Western state of affairs onto other cultures and times.

Ci Cikitsāsthāna/Cikitsitasthāna.
Ka Kalpa(siddhi)sthāna.
Madanamahārṇava *Madanamahārṇava of Śrī Viśveśvara Bhaṭṭa*, ed. Embar Krishnamacharya and M. R. Nambiyar, Gaekwad's Oriental Series 117, (Baroda: Oriental Institute, 1953).
Mādhavanidāna *MahāmatiśrīMādhavakaraviracitaṃ Mādhavanidānam. Mahāmahopādhyāya-śrīVijayarakṣita-Śrīkaṇṭhadattābhyāṃ viracitayā 'Madhukośa'-vyākhyayā vibhūṣitam. Tathā Sudarśanaśāstrikṛtayā 'Vidyotinī' hindīṭīkayā navīnavaijñānika 'Vimarśena' ca samullasitam*, ed. Yadunandanopādhyāya, Kāśī-Saṃskṛta-Granthamālā 158 (Vārāṇasī: Caukhambā Saṃskṛt Sīrīj Āphis, [2]1960–61) (two volumes).
Ni Nidānasthāna.
Śā Śārīrasthāna.
Si Siddhisthāna.
Siddhasāra *The Siddhasāra of Ravigupta. Volume I: The Sanskrit Text*, ed. R. E. Emmerick, Verzeichnis der orientalischen Handschriften in Deutschland, Supplementband 23.1 (Wiesbaden: Franz Steiner Verlag, 1980).
Suśruta. *Suśrutasaṃhitā of Suśruta With the Nibandhasaṅgraha Commentary of Śrī Ḍalhaṇāchārya and the Nyāyacandrikā Pañjikā of Śrī Gayadāsāchārya on Nidānasthāna*, ed. Jādavji Trikamji Āchārya and Nārāyaṇ Rām Āchārya, Jaikrishnadas Ayurveda Series 34 (Varanasi: Chaukhambha Orientalia, [4]1980).
Suśruta[1]. *Sushrut-Sañhitā (Sūtra Sthān) With Bhānumatī Commentary by Chakrapāṇi Datta*, ed. Jādavaji Trikamajī Āchārya and Nandkishor Sharmā Bhishagāchārya, Shrī Swāmī Lakshmī Rām Trust Series 1 ([Jaipur]: Swāmī Lakshmī Rām Trust, 1939).
Sū Sūtrasthāna.
Ut Uttarasthāna/Uttaratantra.
Vi Vimānasthāna.

5

Does Ancient Indian Medicine Have a Theory of Contagion?

Kenneth G. Zysk

When conducting a study of contagion, we must recognize at the outset that it is a theory of disease transmission that derives exclusively from the Western medical tradition. Therefore, we must further be prepared to accept that contagion, understood in Western medicine as a malady caused by "touching" or physical contact, was not or was only incidentally recognized as a source of disease in the medical systems of other cultures, such as ancient India. Further, the boundary between contagion and infection (i.e., disease communicated without physical contact) is blurred in ancient Indian medicine.

In the modern parlance of medical theory, both contagion and infection involve micro-organisms. Ancient Indian medicine focuses primarily on the theories of the origin of diseases and their transmission through means other than physical contact, which certainly do not include micro-organisms. Although the dominant mode of disease transmission was by means other than touching, references to disease causation in the classical texts, and in their later commentarial literature, indicate a recognition that some types of maladies under certain circumstances could be transmitted by physical contact. However, it appears that little significance was placed on this theory of disease transmission. Moreover, the elaboration of the theory occurs first only in an eleventh-century CE commentary, which shows no knowledge of micro-organisms.

My task in this paper is to examine the sources of ancient Indian medicine from the Veda through classical *āyurveda* in order to understand fundamental notions about disease transmission and to isolate any evidence that might point to a recognition of disease communicated by physical contact. Finally, it is useful to compare the ancient Indian medical ideas about disease causation and transmission with those found in the medical traditions of the antique

Western world, so that similarities and differences in roughly contemporaneous ancient medical systems can be seen and provide a potential basis. for further investigations.

Contagion in the Vedic period

Before beginning a discussion of disease transmission in Indian medicine, a brief historical orientation to the literature is helpful. Based on the available literary sources, the history of Indian medicine may be divided into three main phases. The first or Vedic phase dates from about 1200–800 BCE. Information about medicine during this period derives from numerous curative incantations and references to healing found in the Atharvaveda and to a much lesser extent in the *Ṛgveda.* The second or "classical" phase is marked by the advent of the first Sanskrit medical treatises, the *Caraka* and *Suśruta Saṃhitās*, which probably date from a few centuries before to several centuries after the common era. This period includes all subsequent medical treatises dating from before the Muslim invasions of India at the beginning of the eleventh century (these works tend to follow closely the earlier classical compilations). The third of "syncretic" phase is marked by clear influences on the classical paradigm from Islamic or Unānī and other non-classical medical traditions, as witnessed in Bhāvamiśra's sixteenth century work *Bhāvaprakāśa.* The time span for this phase extends from the Muslim incursions to the present era. This threefold division of Indian medical history is simply our working model, providing a convenient orientation to the subject matter.

In the earliest or Vedic phase of Indian medicine, healing may be conceived broadly in terms of magical rituals during which specialized priests exorcised demonic diseases by means of spells and amulets or other apotropaic devices. Except for physical injuries such as broken bones or wounds, diseases were ordinarily considered to have been the result of demonic forces. Indeed, a disease was synonymous with a demon in Vedic India. It was commonly believed that these demons attacked humans as punishment for some sin or evil the human committed, or as a result of a curse cast upon that individual from the work of witchcraft and sorcery. In the minds of the Vedic Indian, disease was either sent by the gods or transmitted by humans via witchcraft or magic. In both instances, disease implied evilness. The usual way to deal with such evil was to remove the demon through exorcism and then to send it away to some distant land or back to its perceived origin. Any reference to contagion or infection is wanting in Vedic medicine. To illustrate Vedic ideas of disease from the Vedic

medical material contained largely in the *Atharvaveda.* These include ascites, consumption (*yakṣma*), *rapas*, dementia, fever (*takman*), *kṣetriya*, leucoderma (*kilāsa*).

Diseases resulting from evil or transgression against the gods

Dropsy, consumption (*yakṣma*), *rapas* and dementia all illustrate the kinds of diseases that the Vedic Indians conceived to be caused by some form of human transgression or evil act committed against a fellow human being or more significantly against a divinity. These maladies, some also demons, attacked humans, but the humans themselves provoked the attacks through their wrongful actions. Ascites or dropsy, known in the Vedic literature as Varuṇa's seizure (*varuṇagṛhīta*), is the disease thought to be sent by a ruling god because of a transgression against the cosmic and moral order (*ṛta*). However, no individual hymns, devoted specifically to this malady, are found. Clear reference to the disease first occurs in the Śunaḥśepa legend of the *Aitareya Brāhmaṇa*, where Varuṇa seized the descendant of Ikṣvāku and his belly swelled up; then with the recitation of the auspicious verses, the bounds around his belly were loosened, his stomach began to shrink, and with the loosing of the last bound, he was released from the seizing-disease. Further references to the morbid bodily state caused by Varuṇa occur in the *Ṛgveda* (7.89.2,4) and the *Atharvaveda* (1.10, 4.16.7, 7.83), where the malady is shown to be sent to a man by Varuṇa because of a transgression against the god and his cosmic order (*ṛta*).[1]

The different passages cited above point to a disease, ascites or dropsy, transmitted to humans by a divine source. The god sent this malady to humans whenever they wronged the god and breached his moral and cosmic law. The disease was specific to Varuṇa and his order, which was considered to include both the moral and natural orders. Whenever an individual transgressed and divinely established order, that person was susceptible to the attack of the god Varuṇa. The disease dropsy was therefore conceived to have been sent to humankind by a ruling god, and each and every case could be attributed to some infringement of the natural laws,including human laws.

One of the most widespread afflictions suffered by the Vedic Indians was *yakṣma*, a type of wasting disease often identified as consumption. It was understood to be a demon or demons that attacked humans of all ages, as well as cattle, and took possession of every part of the victim's body. *Yakṣma* was

[1] See K. G. Zysk, *Medicine in the Veda* (Delhi: Motilal Banarsidass, 1996), 59–61.

known to be sent by the gods as a result of some evil action committed by the victim. The gods sent *yakṣma* for such sinful acts as the dishonest man's pressing of the ritual drink Soma in a sly way, and causing injury to the hairs of a cow.[2] One interesting passage in the famous wedding hymn, parts of which are still used at Hindu weddings, informs us that *yakṣmas* have their origins in the relatives of the bride and that they followed the wedding procession until it was sent back.

> The *yakṣmas* that come from the bride's party follow the glorious wedding procession. May the splendid gods lead them back whence they came.[3]

Although it is only implied, this verse seems to indicate that *yakṣma* was recognized as having been transmitted from humans to humans, perhaps pointing to a simple understanding of hereditary or congenital disease, observed elsewhere in the Veda. The interesting point about this verse is that any form of the malady that afflicted the husband was understood to have originated with the wife and her family. The female was thus the sole transmitter of ill effects on her family and home.

The Vedic Indians understood the demonic disease *rapas* to be an evil entity, divinely sent because of a transgression. It was conceived to be a type of water-borne poison that attacked the limbs and joints, perhaps similar to the known action of the guinea-worm disease.[4] Unlike the previous disease, *rapas* was associated with a specific natural location, i.e., water. Presumably, the transgressor became afflicted with this disease when he entered or came in contact with a body of water. In this way, sinful people were infected by water infested with *rapas*, originally put there by certain divine agents. The transmission was from the gods to humans, but through the intermediary of water. It is entirely possible that Vedic Indians perceived bad or ill-smelling and ill-looking water as fouled and polluted by *rapas*.

---

[2]Ibid., 12–17.

[3]RV 10.85.31. Cf. Louis Renou, trans., *Hymnes spéculatifs du Veda* (Paris: Gallimard, 1956), 87, and his *Études védiques et pāṇinéennes*, Vol. 16, 146. See also Ludwig Alsdorf, *Kleinen Schriften*, ed. by A. Wezler (Wiesbaden: Franz Steiner, 1974), 34–35, K. F. Geldner, trans., *Der Rig-Veda*, Vol. 3 (Cambridge, Mass.: Harvard University Press, 1951), 271, and G. M. Bolling, "Disease and Medicine (Vedic)", in *Encyclopedia of Religion, and Ethics*, Vol. 4, ed. by James Hastings (1912, reprinted New York: C. Scribner's sons, 1955), 769.

[4]See K. G. Zysk, *Medicine in the Veda*, 25–8.

Diseases affecting the mind bridge the gap between the two commonly understood causes of malady in Vedic India, transgression and sorcery. Dementia was conceived to be the state when the mind left the body as a result of a transgression against certain mores or taboos, of an imprecation against the gods, of demonic possession, or of a type of sorcery.[5]

Diseases caused by witchcraft and sorcery

The two demonic entities, *takman* and *Kṣetriya*, illustrate the Vedic diseases that were thought to be caused by witchcraft and sorcery. These demonic forces reveal the Vedic Indians' belief that the power of natural phenomena could be harnessed, controlled, and ultimately transmitted to humans for harmful ends. Destructive power from outside the human body was manipulated and transferred to humans by means of magic. In the case of *kṣetriya*, once inside the human, it was then transmitted to offspring at birth, illustrating again perhaps a simple understanding of hereditary or congenital disease. The spread of such maladies was then from humans to humans.

Takman or fever inside humans, originated from the outside by demonic forces, and then was exorcised and transmitted to other humans as if in an act of warfare. Since there are clear indications that it was a fairly widespread ailment, *takman* became the disease most dreaded by the Vedic Indians.

We know more about the physical effects of the demonic *takman* fever than about its origin. One reference suggests that the fever came from fire, whether from the earth, mid-space or heaven (AV 1.25.1). Most connections occur between the fire of the mid-space, i.e., lightning and the fever demon. The most numerous attacks took place during the seasons of the monsoons. The association between the outbreak of fever and times of the years, indicates a conscious connection between disease and seasons, an equation that is made in ancient Greek and in later classical Indian medicine. We cannot push this observation too far however, because it is merely implied in the various hymns mentioning *takman*. It is clear from the material at our disposal that fever, including most particularly malaria, was a persistent and perennial problem to the Vedic Indians. They dealt with it in the only way they knew—by magic and exorcism. Conceived as a demon, fever could be handled like any other evil entity. With the proper rituals, it was appeased and conquered. Once under the control of the ritualist healer, the fever was expelled from its victims and sent away, far off to its home among the peoples over the mountains, or

---

[5] Ibid., 62–3, 186–8.

to attack other undesirable individuals or enemies. The healer then had the power to eradicate the disease and use it as a weapon to harm others. Just as fever could be used in sorcery to cause injury to others, so, presumably, its attacks on the Vedic people were the result of sorcery connected with the control of fire in its various manifestations.[6]

We can conjecture that the Vedic Indians viewed their most feared disease fever as a demon sent to them by means of witchcraft and sorcery. These evil ritualists manipulated the fires of the mid-space (i.e., lightning) so as to bring about widespread misery during the seasons of heaviest rains. Coming from the outside world, it resulted ultimately from a natural phenomenon (i.e., fire) that was manipulated by means of magic.

Another sorcery-caused malady connected with the environment was the *kṣetriya*, interpreted as a hereditary disease. This demon was associated with the condition of general wasting or consumption, *yakṣma*, which was transmitted from parents to their children. *Kṣetriya* attacked an individual as a result of the ingestion of a mixture concocted with materials from the earth or soil and made harmful by sorcery.[7] Once inside the person, male or female, it was passed on to the offspring, making this demonic disease, like an epidemic, particularly destructive to families and entire clans.

Finally, *kilāsa*, cutaneous white marks or leucoderma on the skin was thought to have been caused by a curse aimed at a particular victim.[8]

In the earliest or Vedic phase of Indian medicine, diseases were generally thought to be of divine origin and were the result of transgressions against the gods or witchcraft and sorcery. This reflects an ideological viewpoint that regarded all evil and misfortune, especially diseases, as a transmission to human beings from the external forces. With the second phase of Indian medicine, an ideological shift in the conception of disease transmission, and indeed of medicine itself, occurred. The Vedic ideas persisted, but they were largely overshadowed by a radically different set of medical presuppositions.

Contagion in classical *āyurveda*

The second or classical phase of Indian medicine is marked by a distinctive change in medical thinking, indicative of an epistemology rooted in empirical

[6] Ibid., 34–44.
[7] See K. G. Zysk, *Medicine in the Veda*, 20–4.
[8] Ibid., 81–2.

observations and reasoning based on a humoral theory.

Central to the classical āyurvedic conception of disease is the theory of the three *doṣas* or defilements, sometimes called humours analogous to the four humours of Hippocratic and Galenic medicine. This theory has no antecedents in Vedic medicine. Simply stated, classical *āyurveda* holds that every disease (*roga, vyādhi*) can be described in terms of the excitement of one or more of the three *doṣas*, wind, bile and phlegm, and of blood, which occasionally takes on the characteristics of a *doṣa*.[9] The defilements themselves are by-products of digested food. When agitated a *doṣa* disrupts the equilibrium between the three, resulting in the manifestation of disease. The derangement of the defilements was thought to be caused by forces either internal or external to the body. Both categories, as we shall see, reveal that diseases can be transmitted from one individual to another or from the environment to humans in the form of epidemics. The "classical" treatises of Caraka and Suśruta discuss these various factors, but it is in Suśruta that we find a classification of diseases based on various internal and external elements that disrupt the balance of the *doṣas*.

Suśruta divides diseases into three types according to their causes: *ādhyātmika*, internally caused diseases; *ādhibhautika*, externally caused diseases; and *ādhidaivika*, divinely or supernaturally caused diseases.[10] These three categories are further classified into types illustrating the range of ways that the early Indian physicians understood disease transmission.

The internally caused diseases include hereditary disease (*ādibala*), congenital diseases (*janmabala*), and humoral diseases (*doṣabala*). The hereditary diseases include, among others, skin diseases and haemorrhoids, and result from defects in the sperm and ovum (*śukraśoṇitadoṣa*) which affect the child. They may derive either from the mother or from the father. Elsewhere, we learn that the defects can be caused by improper postures and practices during coitus.[11]

Congenital diseases include, among others, lameness; congenital blindness, deafness, and dumbness; nasal speech; and dwarfism; and result from an expecting mother's unwholesome conduct. They are said to arise from one or

[9] See G. J. Meulenbeld "The Constraints of Theory in the Evolution of Nosological Classifications: A Study on the Position of Blood in Indian Medicine (Āyurveda)," in G. J. Meulenbeld, ed., *Medical Literature from India, Sri Lanka and Tibet* (Leiden: E. J. Brill, 1991), 91–106; and "Conformities and Divergences of Basic Āyurvedic Society, Vol. 1 (1991), 1–6.

[10] *Suśruta*. Sū 24.4.

[11] *Suśruta*. Sū 2.36–43.

more of the six tastes (*rasa*) and unsatisfied desires or improper conduct of the pregnant woman. Humoral diseases arise form pre-existing morbidities and are caused by improper diet and unwholesome conduct. They can be either gastric or intestinal, which in turn is either physically or mentally caused.[12]

Both the hereditary and congenital disease reflect rather sophisticated notions of human-to-human disease transmission. One takes place at conception, the other during the antenatal stage. Whereas hereditary maladies can be traced back to either the mother or the father, congenital diseases derive solely from the mother as a result of some more impropriety, thus continuing the female source of congenital diseases already found in the Vedic medical tradition. Improper conduct was also the cause of humoral diseases, indicating a strong brahmin religious influence.

Externally caused diseases are traumatic maladies (*saṃghātabala*) such as injuries inflicted on a weaker person by someone or something more powerful. They result either from sharp weapons or from wild beasts.[13] No form of disease transmission is indicated by this category of malady.

Divinely caused diseases result largely from external influences, and include examples that provide the basis for the Indian understanding of epidemics and the spread of malady in the populations.

In this category of disease is found an early reference to maladies communicated by physical contact. Little importance was given to the idea in the early treatises, and the later commentators merely provide examples to help elucidate the text. The Indian physicians recognized that disease could be transmitted by physical contact, but they did not develop a theory of contagion based on their observations.

Divinely caused diseases consist of three types: periodic diseases, i.e., diseases produced from the action of seasons (*kālabala*); providential diseases, i.e., diseases produced from supernatural powers (*daivabala*); and spontaneous diseases, i.e., diseases produced from natural means (*svabhāvabala*). Periodic diseases include as causes, among others, cold and hot winds, rain, and heat, and are produced either by abnormal or normal seasons. Providential diseases result from malice against the gods, from curses, from Atharvaṇa-

[12] *Suśruta*. Sū 24.5. Ḍalhaṇa explains that congenital disease involve abnormalities caused without defilement of the sperm and ovum, and humoral diseases are produced from the power of the humours and of *rajas* and *tamas*. He goes on to say that pre-existing morbidities (*ātaṅka*) refer to disease conditions (*roga*) that are related to one another in what appears to be a kind of symptomatic way, i.e., catarrh causes cough, which causes wasting, etc.

[13] *Suśruta*. Sū 24.6.

magic, or from contact with diseased persons (*upasarga*). They could either come from lightning and thunder or from ghouls, etc., or derive from contact (*saṃsarga*) and by accident (i.e., unperceived means) (*ākasmika*). Finally, spontaneous diseases include, among others, hunger, thirst, old age, death and sleep. They are either timely, i.e., diseases of people who take care of themselves; or untimely (i.e., premature), i.e., diseases of people who do not take care of themselves.[14]

This nosological division of divinely caused disease in particular offers insight into the Indian theory of disease transmission. The Category of providential disease already encountered in the Vedic medical tradition, and therefore, provides a vital link to an older tradition of healing.

Notions about disease caused from contact (*upasarga, saṃsarga*) and by accident (*ākasmika*), however, appear for the first time in the classical medical tradition. It is only with the later commentators Cakrapāṇidatta (eleventh century CE) and Ḍalhaṇa (twelfth century CE), however, that a clear understanding of the key terms *upasarga*, *saṃsarga*, and *ākasmika* begins to emerge. Based largely on Ḍalhaṇa, the word *upasarga* refers to diseases caused by contact with persons afflicted by disease such as fever; the word *saṃsarga* to disease caused by contact with people seeking injury to the gods, etc.; and the word *ākasmika* to diseases produced by the affliction of *karman* (i.e., deeds) in a former life, without contact with people seeking injury to the gods. etc.[15]

Of the two technical Sanskrit words referring to diseases caused by contact, only one, *upasarga*, according to the commentaries actually indicates the transmission of a physical malady by contact. *Saṃsarga* implies a type of supernatural or religious basis for a disease that is communicated through contact with morally tainted persons. The third word discussed in this context, *ākasmika*, has nothing whatsoever to do with the transference of disease by physical contact.

The word *upasarga* is encountered in Suśruta's chapter on the aetiology of skin diseases (*kuṣṭha*) which includes leprosy, where we see clearly a recognition of contagion in its medically literal meaning:

---

[14] *Suśruta*. Sū 24.7. Ḍalhaṇa explains that timely diseases (*kāla*) are those that arrive at the appointed time, and untimely diseases (*akāla*) are those that do not arrive at the appointed time. He goes on to say that timely diseases occur when action is taken to preserve the body, and untimely diseases occur when no action is taken to preserve the body.

[15] Cakrapāṇidatta says that *saṃsarga* refers to diseases caused by contact with infectious, diseased persons; and *ākasmika*, being different from *saṃsarga*, refers to supernaturally caused diseases because it is imperceptible (i.e., unseen).

> Skin disease, fever, consumption, oozing of the eyes (i.e., conjunctivitis), and diseases resulting from contact with a diseased person (*upasarga*) pass from person to person because of [the following]: sexual intercourse [with a diseased person], touching [a diseased person's] body, breathing [near a diseased person], eating from a [diseased person's vessel], sharing [a diseased person's] bed or seat, or using a [diseased person's] clothes, flowery garlands, or unguents.[16]

These references from Suśruta, along with the commentarial remarks, help to provide an understanding of an Indian theory of disease transmitted by human-to-human contact. Given the brāhmaṇic penchant for purity and avoidance of pollution, one would have expected that maladies communicated by physical contact would have received more attention in classical āyurvedic nosology.

What is interesting, however, is Suśruta's mention of skin disease— including leprosy—as contagious. Although shown not to be contagious, leprosy was commonly held by the peoples of the ancient Near East, and more recently of Europe, to be a malady transmitted by physical contact. Could this be a specific example of the exchange of medical information, or is leprosy and other such skin disease universally held to be transmitted by touching? If the former, one might suggest the flow of information was from west to east. Interesting also is Suśruta's inclusion of the condition of oozing of the eyes, generally known as conjunctivitis, as transmitted by physical contact. Today, conjunctivitis is known to be highly contagious.

The use of *karman*, or past deeds, to help explain disease transmission is a uniquely Indian idea and already occurs in this context in the *Caraka Saṃhitā*. Caraka specifies a religious and moral cause for the corruption of wind, water, land, and season, that leads to disease and epidemics.

> Either unrighteousness (*adharma*) or misdeeds in a previous life are the root cause for the corruption of all [the four factors] beginning the wind. Specifically, mistaken judgement is the source

[16] *Suśruta*. Ni 5.33–4. The commentators, Ḍalhaṇa and Gayadāsa (late tenth to early eleventh cent. CE) understand that the primary reference in these verses is to *kuṣṭha* whose chief cause is repeated sexual intercourse with someone afflicted with *kuṣṭha*. Other causes include such a diseased person's touch, breath, etc. In addition, other diseases, such as fever, consumption, etc., are transmitted by the same means. They explain that the diseases resulting from contact with a diseased person (*aupasargikaroga*) are diseases beginning with smallpox (*śītalā*, Ḍalhaṇa; *masūrī*, Gayadāsa).

> of both. As for example—when heads of districts, cities, villages, and nations, after having neglected righteousness (*dharma*), treat their subjects with unrighteousness, then their subordinates and their underlings, both urban and rural people, and businessmen, promote unrighteousness; and because of this, those, whose righteousness is concealed, are forsaken even by the gods. Thus, among these unrighteous people who have hidden away their goodness and who no longer have recourse to the gods, the normal seasonal activities become disturbed. Rains do not arrive at the proper time; they do not come at all; or they fall in abnormal amounts. Winds do not blow properly. Soil erodes. Water reservoirs dry up. Medicinal herbs lose their essential properties and die away. And people are afflicted with epidemics because of the corruption of things with which they come in contact and which they consume.[17]

Moral factors indicative of Brāhmaṇism continue to play a significant role in the medical authors' explanations for the outbreak of diseases, especially large-scale epidemics. These religious elements may form part of what this author has elsewhere called the "Hindu veneer", superimposed on a body of pre-existing medical material.[18]

The effect of the seasons or of the environment in general on the occurrence of disease received attention by both Suśruta and Caraka. In his chapter on the course of the seasons (*ṛtucarya*), Suśruta states that the seasons affect the *doṣas*, and that defects of the seasons cause abnormal food and water, giving rise to the outbreak of various diseases or to an epidemic (*maraka*).[19] He goes on to say that

> Thereupon [there should be] the use of uncorrupted medicinal herbs and water.[20] Sometimes even when the seasons are uncor-

[17] *Caraka*. Vi 3.20. Translation follows Cakrapāṇidatta who explains that the corrupted things one comes in contact with and consumes include bad air, foul odours, as well as food and water. Cf. P. V. Sharma, *Caraka Saṃhitā*, Vol. 3 (Critical Notes) (Varanasi: Chaukhambha Orientalia, 1985), 320–1.

[18] See K. G. Zysk, *Asceticism and Healing in Ancient India* (Delhi, Motilal Banarsidass, 1998).

[19] *Suśruta*. Sū 6.15–17.

[20] *Suśruta*. Sū 6.18. Ḍalhaṇa calls this line a *sūtra* that is concerned with the mishaps from the seasons and points out that some interpret it to mean that "therapy is to be performed with old medicinal herbs that have not lost their potency."

> rupted, people are afflicted by magical actions, curses, the anger of demons, and unrighteousness (*adharma*), Or else, in a region visited by the scent of flowers of poisonous herbs, brought close by the wind, [people suffer], irrespective of humoral balance and physical constitution, from cough, asthma, vomiting, catarrh, headache, and fever. Or else, [they suffer] diseases brought about by the motions of the planets and asterisms, or [by diseases] whose occurrences are caused by portends of a house, wife, bed, seat, vehicle, draught-animal, jewels, gems, or domestic items.[21]

In addition to seasonal and environmental factors, Suśruta includes religious and astrological elements, among those external factors causing disease. The astrological factors are not unique to Indian medicine, and occur, among others, in the antique medical systems of Mesopotamia.

Caraka devotes an entire chapter (Vi 3) to epidemics (*janapadoddhvaṃsanīya*). He discusses the four (environmental) causes of epidemics: wind (*vāta*), water (*jala*), land or place (*deśa*), and time or seasons (*kāla*). He explains that even though people in a particular region may have different physical constitutions, the four factors, when they are corrupted and become abnormal, bring about the simultaneous outbreak of diseases and epidemics.[22]

> Noisome wind does not conform to the seasons. It is excessively moist, stirring, violent, cold, hot, arid, humid, and howling; it all too often blows simultaneously from different directions, impeding each wind's progress, and blows in a whirling motion; and it is charged with noxious odours, vapours, sand, dust, and smoke.
>
> Unclean water is devoid of its usual qualities; and has an exceedingly unnatural smell, colour, taste, and feel; it contains rotting matter; and it is devoid of aquatic birds and fish, and is generally disagreeable.
>
> Insalubrious land has an unnatural colour, smell, taste, and feel. It contains rotting matter, and is infested with snakes, beasts of prey, mosquitoes, locusts, flies, rats, owls, vultures, and jackals; it has thickets of grasses and weeds, and numerous

[21] *Suśruta*. Sū 6.19. Ḍalhaṇa states that this passage speaks about diseases caused by seasons that are not corrupted and explains that unrighteousness (*adharma*) refers to evil action of body, speech and mind. He glossed *upakaraṇa* ("domestic items") as items beginning with a water-jug, pot, and winnowing basket, or else items beginning with a house.

[22] *Caraka*. Vi 3.6.

> tendrilous plants; it has a new appearance; but its crops are uncleared, parched and spoiled, and its air is smoky. Its birds and dogs cry out; its various communities of wild animals and birds are bewildered and agitated; and its people have abandoned righteousness (*dharma*), truthfulness (*satya*), modesty, customs, disciplines, and other merits. Its rivers are constantly agitated and overflowing; and it is overspread with frequent meteor showers, thunderstorms, and earthquakes. It has a fierce and howling appearance. Its sun, moon, and stars are frequently covered over the networks of rough, copper-coloured, ruddy, and white clouds. It appears as if filled with confusion, anxiety, fear, lamentation, and darkness; and is accompanied with sounds of weeping as if frequented by ghoulish (*guhyaka*)-demons.
>
> Unwholesome seasons exhibit signs that are contrary, and either excessive or deficient, to those of the normal seasons.
>
> When these four elements are abnormal, they are the cause of epidemics; but when they are not, they are wholesome. When properly treated with (prophylactic) medicaments, people do not succumb to disease, even when these four environmental factors are defiled.[23]

Both Caraka and Suśruta also recognize that diet, as an external factor, contributes to disease. Suśruta explains,

> The imprudent person who consumes [substances] incompatible in taste and potencies experiences disease, debility of the sense organs, or death. Disease is caused when the substance consumed, after having made a humour move from its seat, is not eliminated for the body, or when it is incongruous with the tastes, etc.[24]

In the classical phase of Indian medicine, as represented in the medical compendia of Caraka and Suśruta, an aetiology appears which utilized the concept of bodily defilements (*doṣas*) that could disrupt the biology of an organism and cause diseases. Likewise, there emerged, in part at least from empirical observation, an understanding of a relationship between human beings and their environment. In this connection, certain environmental factors acted upon individual or people, causing diseases and epidemics. Moreover,

[23] *Caraka*. Vi 3.7–8.

[24] *Suśruta*. Sū 20.19–20; see also *Caraka*. Sū 25.31.

some maladies were known to be transferable from individual to individual by physical contact, providing the basis for an Indian theory of disease transmission by touch. This early Indian idea of "contagion", however, seems to have played an insignificant role in the overall systems of Indian nosology. Finally, as a carryover from the earlier Vedic medical tradition, different supernatural powers acted as causers of disease. The combination of these elements in classical Indian medicine reveal it to have a sophisticated system of disease transmission in antiquity.

Ancient Indian and Greek notions of contagion compared

It is useful at this point to compare briefly the ancient Indian ideas of the transmission of diseases with those of the ancient world in the West.[25] Like the ancient Indian physicians, the ancient Greek doctors focused on the causation and transmission of diseases, and paid little attention to specific theories of contagion and infection as they were to be known later in the Western traditions. In fact, it would be safe to say that the precursor of these forms of disease transmission is not to be found among the medical traditions of the Hellenistic period.[26]

One of the central ideas of disease transmission in Hippocratic, as in classical Indian, medicine, involved environmental factors. The Hippocratics developed the theory of miasma or bad air, i.e., air polluted by noxious vapours, to explain the outbreak of widespread diseases in a region of regions. In the Hippocratic writings miasmic theory was based on observations of the effects of natural phenomena, such as climate and season, and of locality on the outbreak of epidemics. These factors produced a miasma that resulted from "a defilement of the air, due to some mysterious agents suspended in it"; and epidemics came about because of the presence of the miasma.[27]

Galen expanded the notion of miasma or defiled air to include an energizing spirit, i.e., pneuma, that the body absorbs from the atmosphere. Explaining Galen's contribution to the notion of miasma, Michael Dols states:

---

[25]The important works on contagion in the Western medical tradition are Oswei Tempkin, *The Double Face of Janus* (Baltimore: Johns Hopkins University Press, 1977), 456–71; Vivian Nutton, "The Seeds of Disease. An Explanation of Contagion and Infection from the Greeks to the Renaissance," *Medical History*, 27 (1983), 1034; and Michael W. Dols, *Medieval Islamic Medicine. Ibn Riḍwān's Treatise "On the Prevention of Bodily Ills in Egypt"* (Berkeley: University of California Press, 1984).

[26]See in this context, the paper of Vivian Nutton in this collection.

[27]See Dols, *Medieval Islamic Medicine*, 18, and Tempkin, *The Double Face of Janus*, 458–9.

> In this view, epidemic disease resulted from the assimilation of vital air fouled by putrid exhalations of decaying matter, such as unburied corpses or swamps and stagnant waters in summertime. Decay or putrescence of organic bodies—*sepsis*,... was the source of pollution, and its evil smell was an indication of and a guide to its prevalence. The noxious miasma might be carried by the wind from distant areas where putrefaction was in progress. A warm, moist air charged with corruption might brood over a stricken land and affect all living things; among susceptible human beings it caused epidemics.[28]

Even more important to Galen than the condition of the air was the internal state of the human body in acquiring a particular disease during an epidemic.[29] In Hippocratic and Galenic medicine, the process of disease transmission resulted from a defiled environment, most often from polluted air. Galen also recognized that an individual's physical state contributed to his or her susceptibility to disease. Hellenistic medicine generally viewed disease as transmitted to humans from the outside. Transference of disease from humans to humans, although perceived, was, as Vivian Nutton points out, not taken seriously.[30]

When we compare these Greek ideas of disease aetiology with those of the Indians, we find that both shared a fundamental belief in the importance of environmental factors in the causation of disease. Similarly, in addition to bad air, both traditions recognized foul water as the source of disease.

Moreover, Caraka's isolation and discussion of the four environmental factors of wind, water, land, and time (i.e., season) in relationship to epidemics bear a conceptual similarity to basic ideas presented the Hippocratic *Airs, Waters, Places,* the fundamental principles of which are outlined in the opening passage.

> Whoever wishes to pursue properly the science of medicine must proceed thus. First he ought to consider what effects each **season** of the year can produce; for the seasons are not at all alike, but differ widely both in themselves and at their changes. The next point is the hot **winds** and the cold, especially those that

[28] Dols, *Medieval Islamic Medicine,* 18.
[29] Ibid, 19.
[30] Nutton, "Seeds of Disease," 6–8.

> are universal, but also those that are peculiar to each particular **region**. He must consider the properties of the **waters**; for as these differ in taste and in weight, so the property of each is far different from that of any other. Therefore, on arrival at a town with which he is unfamiliar, a physician should examine its position with respect to the winds and to the risings of the sun. For a northern, a southern, an eastern, and a western aspect has each its own individual property. He must consider with the greatest of care both these things and how the natives are off for water, whether they use marshy, soft waters, or such as are hard and come from rocky heights, or brackish and harsh. The **soil** too, whether bare or dry or wooded and watered, hollow and hot or high and cold. The mode of life also of the inhabitants that is pleasing to them, whether they are heavy drinkers, taking lunch, and inactive, or athletic, industrious, eating and drinking little.[31]

The Hippocratic writer, likewise, isolates seasons, winds, waters, land (region and soil) as the four environmental factors crucial to understanding the health, disease, and outbreak of epidemics in a place.

In addition to the environmental factors, the Greek physicians, like their Indian counterparts, recognized that lifestyle also contributed to peoples' state of health or disease. However, where the Greeks stressed the physical way of life, the Indian's emphasized the moral and religious mode of life practised in a region, even bringing in the pan-Indian idea of past deeds or *karman* as contributing to disease and epidemics.

These few examples from the early Greek medical literature provide explanations of disease causation similar to those found in the classical Indian medical treatises. Moreover, common to each system was a humoral-based theory and the disruption of the balance of humours created by the environment. Religion, in the form of correctness of character and action, also played a part in philosophy of disease causation among the Indians. The Greeks, on the other hand, downplayed the importance of religion in the occurrence and transmission of diseases, preferring to attribute the cause of certain widespread maladies to the lifestyle of the inhabitants of a given area. Neither ancient tradition provides explanations of contagion and infection exactly in

---

[31] W. H. S. Jones, trans. Hippocrates. Vol. 1 (Cambridge, Mass.: Harvard University Press, 1972), 71–3 [Loeb Classical Library]. I have put words in bold type.

terms they are understood today, but both handled the causation and transmission of disease, and their characteristics in very similar ways.

While it is admittedly difficult to isolate any one-to-one correspondence between ancient Greek and Indian medicine, there clearly exist certain conceptual similarities, particularly in the area of disease causation and transmission. Are these similarities simply coincidental or do they suggest a closer relationship between the two systems than previously thought? In order to answer this question, which has nagged historians of ancient medical systems for over a century, further research is obviously required. Hopefully this piece and others in this volume will contribute to further inquiry into these two ancient medical systems and the possible relationship between them.

Part III

MIDDLE EAST and EUROPE

6

OLD TESTAMENT "LEPROSY", CONTAGION AND SIN

Elinor Lieber

The term contagion is often applied to any form of transmission of a communicable disease but, strictly speaking, it indicates the spread of an illness by direct or indirect contact and here it will be considered in that sense. Other contributions to this volume show that many ancient peoples possessed some idea of these concepts. As regards ancient Judaism, the Old Testament frequently alludes to the sudden infliction of "pestilences" and epidemics by God; but it is not at all clear whether the victims were struck down individually, or if the outbreak spread from person to person. However, while presenting few helpful details on acute epidemics, the Hebrew Bible provides more information regarding certain chronic endemic diseases, although here too, any references to physical contagion are only rarely specific. One exception is the description in Leviticus 15:2–13 of a man with a genito-urinary discharge.[1] Again, it seems clear from Numbers 19:11–16 that the "uncleanness" arising from contact with a corpse is due to the fear of contagion. In general, however, the existence of such a concept can only be determined indirectly.

This is particularly the case with reference to the Biblical *ṣāra'at*, a term that, in various forms, appears 35 times throughout the Hebrew Old Test-

In memory of my dermatology teacher, Dr. J. Randell Vickers, 1914–93. I gratefully acknowledge the assistance of Professor T. J. Ryan, of the Randell Vickers Dermatology Department, Churchill Hospital, Oxford. An earlier version of this paper gained the 14th Samuel J. Zakon Award in the History of Dermatology, 1992, presented by the U.S. History of Dermatology Society.

[1] Cf. the very similar non-Biblical injunctions, from around 1700 BC, regarding a sick woman in Mesopotamia. See R. Briggs, "Medicine in Ancient Mesopotamia," *History of Science* 8 (1969): 94–105. However, although in Leviticus 15 a man suffering from such a discharge must be isolated as long as the condition persists, in vv. 16–18 this is contrasted with a simple ejaculation, for which the man is only "unclean" the same day.

ament.[2] It generally refers to certain skin conditions in man, although, according to Leviticus 13:47–59 and 14:33–55, it also concerns garments and houses. In fact, only the *ṣāra'at* of houses is unequivocally described as contagious (Leviticus 14:46–7). In modern Hebrew, *ṣāra'at* is not used as a medical term. Its meaning and derivation are uncertain,[3] but it may be related to the Akkadian *saḫaršubbû*, which refers to some disease that "covers" the skin with white "dust" and is now usually translated as "leprosy".[4]

In the Septuagint, dating from the third century BC, *ṣāra'at* is rendered as *lepros*, which later passed to the Vulgate as *lepra*, both denoting "scaly", "scabby", or "rough". Yet, from its Biblical contexts, the Hebrew term seems to indicate some dreaded disease. Hence in almost every subsequent translation of the Bible *ṣāra'at* has been interpreted as "leprosy" (or its equivalent in other languages). Until quite recent times this was generally considered to indicate true leprosy (Hansen's disease), even though this condition affects neither garments nor houses.

However, according to Rufus of Ephesus, around AD 100, a disease named *elephantiasis* had been described some five centuries earlier by Straton, an Alexandrian Greek. From the accounts of the condition provided by Rufus himself and by his contemporary, Aretaeus of Cappadocia, this seems very like modern lepromatous leprosy, the most severe form of the disease.[5] The latter attributes the Greek appellation to the elephant-like changes produced by the disease, such as fissuring of the skin. The (ps.-) Galenic *Introductio seu*

---

[2]See T. Seidl, art. "Ṣāra'at" in *Theologisches Wörterbuch zum Alten Testament*, ed. G. J. Botterweck, H. Ringgren, and H. J. Fabry (Stuttgart: Kohlhammer, 1989), VI, 1127–9.

[3]See J. F. A. Sawyer, "A Note on the Etymology of *Ṣāra'at*," *Vetus Testamentum* 26 (1976): 241–5; Seidl, "Ṣāra'at", 1127–9.

[4]*Assyrian Dictionary*, XV (Chicago: University of Chicago, 1984), *s.v.*; J. V. Kinnier Wilson, "Leprosy in Ancient Mesopotamia," *Revue d'assyriologie* 60 (1966): 47–58; Briggs, "Medicine in Ancient Mesopotamia," 94. However, according to an inscription quoted by A. L. Oppenheim, "The Interpretation of Dreams in the Ancient Near East," *Transactions of the American Philosophical Society*, New Series, 46 (1956): 273, n. 54, the term is applied to a "leper" covered with a white scaly dust. If so, as will be seen, it would probably refer to a case of chronic psoriasis.

[5]For Rufus, see Oribasius, *Collectionum medicarum reliquiae* 45.28, *CMG*, VI.ii.1, ed. J. Raeder (Berlin: Teubner, 1930), III, 184; *Aretaeus* IV.13, ed. C. Hude, *CMG*, II, 2nd ed. (Berlin: Akademie Verlag, 1958), 85–90. From around the same period, and also under the name "elephantiasis", the Roman author Celsus provides a brief but accurate description of leprosy in his *De medicina* III.25.1–2; Loeb trans. by W. G. Spencer (London: Heinemann, 1960–1), I, 342. Here leprosy is not confused with filariasis (a totally different disease; see n. 6 below), as the translator maintains (I, 342 n. a).

medicus (XIV, 757–8 Kühn) refers to the "elephantine" appearance of the legs, or "woody oedema", which is still considered as an early sign of leprosy.[6]

True leprosy is a chronic, progressive, bacterial infection.[7] Contrary to much modern dogma, in its common "low resistance" or lepromatous form it is contagious, although not all those affected present macroscopic signs of the condition. The infectivity of untreated cases depends on the stage of the disease and on the degree of contact with others. Individual predisposition, due to genetic and other familial factors, also plays a role. Death usually occurs from some secondary infection, often many years after the sufferer first becomes aware of the disease.

The contagious skin lesions, which constitute one of the earliest manifestations of lepromatous leprosy, are not only apparent to the sufferer but may also be noticed by others. They include hypopigmented areas that often appear whitish or white,[8] although any hair in the lesion is not affected in this way. The skin becomes thickened, fissured and wrinkled, and raised nodules, or lepromata, appear over the body, particularly on the face and the ears. Typically, the skin of the forehead is thickened and the eyebrows are lost. While the skin lesions may ulcerate, the main means of spread is probably airborne infection from early involvement of the interior of the nose. Later, the nose and upper jaw may be destroyed, thus producing the terrible dis-

---

[6]W. H. Jopling, *Handbook of Leprosy*, 3rd ed. (London: Heinemann, 1984), 20. Hence, leprosy was then usually known as *elephantiasis graecorum*, thus distinguishing it from the infestation by certain tropical filarial worms, which also causes gross swelling of the legs. However, in modern medicine the term elephantiasis refers essentially to the latter condition.

According to Aretaeus (*loc. cit.*), true leprosy was also known as *elephas* in Greek; but if, as seems likely, the term was also used to denote filarial elephantiasis, the latter might be represented by the very similar Hebrew term *yalefet*, a hitherto unidentified condition mentioned in Leviticus 21:20, 22:22. In the Talmud (*Bekhorot* VI, 12; 41a) this is said to denote some condition found in Egypt, where filariasis of all kinds is prevalent indeed. The Bible provides no description of *yalefet*, which is translated in the Septuagint as *leichēn*. In this paper (see below) the latter, in other contexts, is identified with a condition known in Arabic as bejel, which also is present in Egypt.

[7]See R. G. Cochrane and T. F. Davey, eds., *Leprosy in Theory and Practice*, 2nd ed. (Bristol: Wright, 1964), *passim*; J. Convit and M. Ulrich, "Recent Advances in the Immunology of Leprosy," *International Journal of Dermatology* 15 (1976): 157–70; D. S. Ridley, *Pathogenesis of Leprosy* (London: Wright, 1988), *passim*; O. Canizares, R. Harman, and B. Adriaans in O. Canizares and R. R. M. Harman, eds., *Clinical Tropical Dermatology*, 2nd ed. (Oxford: Blackwell, 1992), 165–200.

[8]See, for example, the illustrations in R. H. Champion, J. L. Burton, and F. J. G. Ebling, eds., *(Rook's) Textbook of Dermatology*, 5th ed. (Oxford: Blackwell, 1992), II, 1075 Fig. 25.20, 1080 Fig. 25.26.

figurement known as a *leonine facies* (*leontiasis*), which from very early times has been considered as typifying true leprosy. The nerves are affected, but the resultant cutaneous anaesthesia, a well-known symptom of leprosy, may only appear late in the disease, as is the case with the highly visible deformities of the limbs. Other common, serious sequelae are sterility and lagophthalmos, which is often followed by blindness.

Yet, since the condition is usually well-established before its distinguishing features appear, leprosy can easily be confused with other chronic endemic diseases. In the Near and Middle East it must be differentiated above all from bejel (endemic treponematosis), from diffuse cutaneous leishmaniasis and, in its early stages, even from the non-contagious skin lesions of vitiligo and chronic psoriasis. Bejel and leishmaniasis will be considered below. The last two conditions are common worldwide and probably always have been so.

In vitiligo (leucoderma),[9] hypopigmented light or white patches appear on the skin, but unlike psoriasis, the lesions are not scaly. Moreover, unlike both psoriasis and leprosy, or any other common condition, the hair in the lesions may turn white. Unless it serves as an indicator of some underlying generalized disease, it is simply a "cosmetic" disorder. This is a perfectly innocuous condition, but the unsightly lesions can cause psychological distress, as in the much publicized case of the black entertainer, Michael Jackson.

Although in chronic psoriasis the commonest signs appear in the skin, it is a systemic condition and may give rise to arthritis and other severe manifestations. However, none of the lesions are contagious, except in the rare cases when secondary infection occurs. In its typical form the skin becomes roughened by scaly, raised, white plaques or "scabs" on a salmon-pink base, particularly on the limbs and the scalp. The scales are characteristically shiny and silvery-white. The disease usually persists throughout life, in the form of attacks that spontaneously remit after a variable period of time. The sufferer may then appear to be "cured", but eventually the skin lesions reoccur. They are more disfiguring than those of vitiligo and may cause even greater distress to the sufferer. In the popular mind psoriasis has always been held to be contagious, probably due to its unsightly skin lesions, which may periodically discharge into the air showers of whitish scales (or "dust", corresponding with

[9]The condition was clearly described by Celsus (*De medicina* V.28.18B; trans. Spencer, II, 172) under the name *leuce*, which he considered as one form of "*vitiligo*". For a modern description, see P. E. Grimes, art. "Vitiligo" in *Andrews' Diseases of the Skin*, 8th ed., ed. R. B. Odom, W. D. James, and H. L. Arnold *et al.* (Philadelphia: Saunders, 1990), 1000–3.

the Akkadian expression noted above), which might be thought to "contaminate" other persons and objects. Such assumptions only add to the expressions of disgust and rejection directed at the unfortunate sufferers. Nothing is known of the cause of the condition, but familial and hereditary elements play a part, and the attacks may be triggered by psychological factors.[10]

Psoriasis in its turn is often associated and confused with other relatively harmless "rough" and "scaly" skin conditions, such as various types of eczema and seborrheic dermatitis, even though in these cases the scales are neither silvery nor bright. Hence the latter may be included in ancient descriptions of skin lesions that seem otherwise consistent with psoriasis.

Clearly, the terms *lepros* and *lepra* do not specifically refer to true leprosy. The (ps.-) Galenic *Introductio* defines *lepra* only as a condition in which the skin is white and rough, and in general these terms would more accurately apply to certain types of eczema and particularly to chronic psoriasis.[11]

It is now similarly maintained that the criteria of Leviticus 13 do not correspond with the manifestations of leprosy, at least as we know it today. This conclusion is largely based on the mistaken assumptions that its lesions are never white and that those of *ṣāra'at* are described as "white as snow" (see n. 29 below). However, it has also rightly been noted that leprosy does not turn the hair white; that cutaneous anaesthesia and other pathognomonic signs of leprosy are not mentioned in the Bible; and that, unlike *ṣāra'at* (see Leviticus 14:3), this condition could not be "cured" in the past.[12]

In addition, the idea still prevails that true leprosy was not present in the Middle East or Egypt before the fourth century BC, but was possibly brought there by Alexander the Great on returning from his Indian campaign. As discussed in some detail below, it has lately been suggested, however, that the disease was present in Mesopotamia and perhaps even in Egypt from very

---

[10] On psoriasis, see P. D. Mier and P. C. M. van de Kerkhof, *Textbook of Psoriasis* (Edinburgh: Churchill Livingstone, 1986), esp. 84–90; H. H. Roenigk Jr. and H. I. Maibach, eds., *Psoriasis*, 2nd ed. (New York: Dekker, 1991).

[11] See F. S. Glickman, "Lepra, Psora, Psoriasis," *Journal of the American Academy of Dermatology* 14 (1986): 863–6. However, in certain parts of the world, such as northern Italy, *lepra* may have indicated pellagra (= "rough skin"). In this serious generalized disease, which is due to a vitamin deficiency, the skin becomes very rough but not white.

[12] K. P. C. A. Gramberg, " 'Leprosy' and the Bible," *The Bible Translator* 11 (1960): 10–23; Y. Tas, "Contagion of *Tsaraat*," in *Encyclopaedia Biblica* (Hebrew) (Jerusalem: Mosad Bialik, 1971), VI, cols. 776–8; L. Koehler and W. Baumgartner, *Hebraeisches und Aramaeisches Lexicon zum Alten Testament*, 3rd ed. (Leiden: Brill, 1990), IV, *s.v. Tsāra'at*; J. Cule, letter in *Journal of the Royal Society of Medicine* 80 (1987): 534.

early times.[13] This has strengthened the minority view, which has always existed, that the term *ṣāra'at* applies *essentially* to true leprosy (with or without other lesser diseases).[14]

Even so, on the accumulated evidence, including the lack of palaeopathological findings, it is now generally assumed that true leprosy is not indicated in the Biblical *ṣāra'at*, or at most plays a very minor role.[15] Yet, surprisingly enough, it has hardly ever been suggested that the term might also, or even alternatively, cover some other major disease.[16] In fact, the interpretation of the *ṣāra'at* of objects (Leviticus 13:47–59) as some kind of "contagious" fungal infestation is perhaps the only "medical" identification on which there is now a consensus.[17]

Hence, even those who accept that the signs of *ṣāra'at* serve to indicate actual diseases now tend to consider this concept as solely of "ritual" or "cultic" significance. The "ritual impurity" was based not on the infliction of leprosy or any other dreaded contagious disease, but on the presence of some relatively

---

[13]On the early history of leprosy, see M. D. Grmek, *Diseases in the Ancient Greek World*, trans. M. and L. Muellner (Baltimore: Johns Hopkins, 1989), 152–76.

[14]Ibid., 161. According to *Julius Preuss' Biblical and Talmudic Medicine* [1911], ed. and trans. F. Rosner (New York: Sanhedrin Press, 1978), 326–7, *ṣāra'at* "probably" refers to "leprosy", considered as a "collective name" comprising three forms: "spotty" (i.e. patchy), nodular, and "psoriasis or... *lepra vulgaris*". Such a classification is no longer valid in medicine today.

[15]See n. 12 above; also E. V. Hulse, "The Nature of Biblical 'Leprosy'," *Palestine Exploration Quarterly* 107 (1975): 87–105; S. G. Browne, *Leprosy in the Bible*, 3rd ed. (London: Christian Medical Fellowship, 1979), 6; M. W. Dols, "Leprosy in Medieval Arabic Medicine," *Journal of the History of Medicine* 34 (1979): 314–33; J. G. Anderson, "Leprosy in Translations of the Bible," *Bible Translator* 31 (1980): 207–12; G. M. Beitman, "Sara'at, 'Leprosy' (Leviticus 13)," *Koroth* 9 (1991): 818–25.

[16]One exception is S. Muntner in F. Rosner, *Medicine in the Bible and Talmud* (New York: Yeshiva University Press, 1977), 11, who suggests *ulcus durum penis* (the venereal "hard chancre") in Leviticus 13:43 (the Hebrew term here for "flesh" can also mean "penis"), "leishmaniasis" (Leviticus 13:42), "chronic syphilis (yaws *et al.*)" (Leviticus 13:11), but provides no further explanations.

[17]See, for example, G. R. Driver, R. G. Cochrane, and H. Gordon, art. "Leprosy" in *Dictionary of the Bible*, 2nd ed., ed. J. Hastings, F. C. Grant, and H. H. Rowley (Edinburgh: Clark, 1963), 575–8; but especially R. Schoental, letter in *Journal of the Royal Society of Medicine* 81 (1988): 58, although one can hardly agree with her conclusion that the undoubtedly toxic and carcinogenic nature of these moulds had already been recognized by the ancient Hebrews. However, as this is a spreading condition, it might well have been considered as "contagious".

harmless non-contagious skin conditions, such as eczema, vitiligo, scabies or psychosomatic disorders and above all, of chronic psoriasis.[18]

It has been further suggested that such lesions, particularly those of psoriasis, were categorized as *ṣāra'at* since, although quite innocuous, they are "scaly" or "flaky" and therefore "repulsive", and thus were considered "unclean".[19] Such lesser conditions would hardly account for the stringent provisions of Leviticus 13–14, and some do not even match the Biblical criteria. Thus, it was already long ago claimed by a doyen of modern dermatology that the term *ṣāra'at* referred "not to a particular disease—certainly not leprosy—but rather to a special kind of uncleanness," a "taboo". The mark on the skin simply represented a recognizable "token of God's wrath", imposed "as punishment for some secret sin of the subject".[20]

Recently this theory has been given a new twist. It has been suggested that since isolation for *ṣāra'at* was decreed only for "moral contagion", the signs given in Leviticus 13 were intentionally made to fit no known disease, in order to exclude those whose only sin was to be affected by "an obvious cutaneous disease".[21] According to another variant theory, in Leviticus 13 the term *ṣāra'at*:

> is applied to various skin diseases... which sooner rather than later may break out into open sores. It is this running sore with the naked blood that makes these skin diseases ritually unclean.

---

[18] For scabies, see n. 42 below; "a neurodermatitis primarily due to psychic tension... aided by the trauma and dirt of rural and agricultural life:" M. Lloyd Davies and T. A. Lloyd Davies, "Biblical Leprosy, a Comedy of Errors," *Journal of the Royal Society of Medicine* 82 (1989): 622; mainly psoriasis: Hulse, "The Nature of Biblical 'Leprosy'," 98; ringworm of the scalp (tinea): F. C. Lendrum, "The Name 'Leprosy'," *American Journal of Tropical Medicine and Hygiene* 1 (1952): 999–1008.

[19] Hulse, "The Nature of Biblical 'Leprosy'." Yet it has long been noted, as in *A Dictionary of the Bible*, ed. W. Smith (London: Murray, 1861–3), II, *s.v.* "Leper," that the Hebrew Leviticus makes no mention of scaling or peeling as a sign of either *ṣāra'at* or "uncleanness". Despite this, the term "scale-disease", suggested by Hulse, has been adopted by a number of Biblical scholars, e.g. J. Milgrom, trans., *Leviticus 1–16, The Anchor Bible* (New York: Doubleday, 1991), 768.

[20] P. G. Unna, "An Exemplary Instance of Faulty Scholarship" [1912] (trans. and abridged), *American Journal of Dermatopathology* 5 (1983): 569–74. See also the informal report to dermatologists on the interim conclusions of an international interfaith committee on revisions of the Bible: L. Goldman, R. S. Moraites, and K. W. Kitzmiller, "White Spots in Biblical Times," *Archives of Dermatology* 93 (1966): 744–53.

[21] D. L. Kaplan, "Biblical Leprosy: an Anachronism Whose Time has Come," *Journal of the American Academy of Dermatology* 28 (1993): 507–10.

> Whether they are medically contagious or not is not the point at issue; what matters here is that they are ritually contagious. The resultant contagion is ritual not medical.[22]

However, all the assumptions of this kind lead to a common conclusion: that any "hygienic" or "public health" consequences of the Biblical rulings can simply be dismissed as a "by-product".[23]

Due to these multiple and often conflicting opinions, many recent translations of the Bible continue to render *ṣāraʿat* as "leprosy", although generally with the proviso that this term refers to various skin diseases, among which true leprosy may or may not be included.[24] In view of this ambiguous status, the Hebrew term will be retained in this paper.

The many Biblical references to *ṣāraʿat* are rarely detailed enough to allow of any serious consideration of the term. The few actual descriptions of the condition are found in two quite different contexts. In certain accounts, designated here as "case histories", it is associated with named persons, but its legal and spiritual connotations are mainly confined to Leviticus 13–14, where its presence is associated with notions of "uncleanness" or "impurity". With such diverse aspects the literature on the subject is vast.[25]

---

[22]N. H. Snaith, ed., *The Century Bible: Leviticus and Numbers*, new ed. (London: Nelson, 1967), 92.

[23]For example, by Hulse in his "The Nature of Biblical 'Leprosy'," 94; K. Elliger, art. "Leviticus" in *Handbuch zum Alten Testament*, IV (Tübingen: Mohr, 1966), 181. On the other hand, A. Rendle Short, *The Bible and Modern Medicine* (London: Paternoster Press, 1953), 77–80, even considers that Leviticus 13 describes true leprosy and yet (in order to promote the humane treatment of leprosy today) maintains that the Biblical exclusion "was not for fear of infection but primarily for religious reasons."

[24]As by Elliger, "Leviticus," 180. Others employ or suggest euphemisms, such as "skin disease": L. Koehler, "Aussatz," *Zeitschrift für die Alttestamentliche Wissenschaft* 67 (1955): 290–1; "a leprous disease on the skin of his body:" *The New Oxford Annotated Bible*, ed. B. M. Metzger and R. E. Murphy (New York: Oxford University Press, 1991), Leviticus 13:2; or the totally inappropriate "malignant skin disease": *The New English Bible with the Apocrypha* (Oxford: Oxford University Press, 1970), Leviticus 13:2.

[25]For a brief selection of general reviews, see Preuss, *Biblical and Talmudic Medicine*, 323–39; R. K. Harrison, art. "Leprosy" in *The Interpreter's Dictionary of the Bible* (Nashville: Abingdon Press, 1962–76), III, 111–13; Driver, "Leprosy;" Elliger, "Leviticus," 159–91; R. Brown, art. "Leprosy (in the Bible)" in *New Catholic Encyclopedia* (New York: McGraw Hill, 1967), VIII, 667–70; H. Michman, art. "Leprosy" in *Encyclopaedia Judaica*, XI (Jerusalem: Keter, 1971), cols. 33–6; Grmek, *Diseases*, 152–76; T. Seidl, *Tora für den "Aussatz"-Fall* (St. Ottilien: EOS Verlag, 1982), 245–53; *idem.*, "Ṣāraʿat," 1127–34.

While the "case histories" have of course frequently been considered with regard to the meaning of *ṣāraʿat*, they have rarely been treated as a whole and certainly not in great detail. Most contributions deal essentially with the relevant text of Leviticus and view the subject as a question of religious belief. In this study, however, the relationship of *ṣāraʿat* to contagion will be examined as widely as possible, using the "case histories" on the one hand and the moral and legal precepts on the other. Yet any attempt to interpret the Biblical text in this manner is hampered by the concise nature of its descriptions in general and by difficulties regarding the interpretation of ancient medical terms. Nor is the task rendered easier by the fact that the Bible is not a medical work and that Leviticus—our main source regarding *ṣāraʿat*—forms part of the Pentateuch and thus essentially deals with the law.

When adopting this point of view, one must take into consideration not only the limitations of ancient medical knowledge, but also the very different concepts of disease in past times and hence the purpose of "diagnosis" as such. The divergences were not necessarily due to lack of medical knowledge in the past, for indigenous concepts were sometimes better attuned than our own to the problems occurring at some far-distant period and place.[26]

Old Testament "case histories" of *ṣāraʿat*

Numbers 12 provides one of the fullest accounts of persons afflicted by *ṣāraʿat*. It is based on material originating at the period of the Exodus from Egypt, when the Israelites were wandering in the desert. Miriam first "speaks out about"[27] the Cushite (non-Jewish) wife of her brother Moses.[28] She and Aaron then claim that God had not "spoken" solely with Moses, but had also "spoken" with them (v. 2). Here they seem to express their jealousy of the

[26] Since the latter observation applies to all post-Biblical views on *ṣāraʿat*, these have largely been omitted in this study, except in the Epilogue below.

[27] Unless otherwise stated, all the Biblical citations here are literal translations by the author of this paper, based on the *Biblia Hebraica Stuttgartensia*, ed. K. Elliger and W. Rudolph, 2nd ed. (Stuttgart: Deutsche Bibelgesellschaft, 1984).

[28] According to the Babylonian Talmud (*Arakhin* IIIv;16b), *ṣāraʿat* may be inflicted for seven sins, including *lashon ha-raʿ*, "speaking ill" of someone, but no reference is made there to Miriam. This term is still widely interpreted as "slander", which is then considered as the sin for which Miriam was punished. See Preuss, *Biblical and Talmudic Medicine*, 337; J. Neuberger, "The History and Management of AIDS: a Biblical and Jewish View," *International Journal of STD and AIDS* 2, Supplement 1 (1991): 34–7. Yet Miriam's outspokenness was not "slander", since, even if her criticism were maliciously intended, as far as we know it was true.

relationship of Moses to God and even question God's choice of intermediary. In any case, God "suddenly" appeared and reproached them, whereupon Miriam found herself afflicted with *ṣāra'at* "like snow" (vv. 4–10).[29]

In the past this was held to indicate that Miriam was inflicted with true leprosy,[30] but insofar as her condition is accepted as a physical disease, it is now generally thought to allude to some non-contagious and far less serious condition: perhaps vitiligo, but probably chronic psoriasis. It has been plausibly suggested that the Biblical comparison of *ṣāra'at* with snow is based not on the actual lesions of psoriasis, but on its typical shiny white scales, which are so copiously shed. For since snow in the Middle East is usually a fleeting phenomenon, this term would there evoke the snow falling as white flakes, rather than in the form of a white covering.[31] If so, Miriam's *ṣāra'at* cannot be considered as vitiligo, which, not being scaly, would hardly have been likened to snow.

If this were an attack of psoriasis, it could well have been triggered by guilt and fear when, after showing lack of faith in God's judgement, Miriam was "suddenly" confronted by God (v. 4). Moreover, there is a hereditary element in psoriasis, and Moses is said to have been similarly affected when his faith in God began to waver (Exodus 4:6–7).[32] Thus, both Moses and Aaron would

[29]The Hebrew of this simile, here and elsewhere in the Bible, is often wrongly rendered in English as "white as snow", as noted by J. L. Swellengrebel, "Leprosy and the Bible," *The Bible Translator* 11 (1960): 69–80, among others.

[30]As still, for example, by Snaith, *Leviticus and Numbers*, 236, who considers that "like snow" means "an open wound or ulcer", as in the description of "leprosy" in Leviticus 13.

[31]Hulse, "The Nature of Biblical 'Leprosy'," 92–3. See also n. 4 above.

[32]Genesis 30:35–42 demonstrates that the ancient Israelites possessed some empirical knowledge of the laws of heredity, at least as concerns animal husbandry.

Exodus 4 deals with the first lone sojourn of Moses on a mountain, when his faith in God was repeatedly tested. While clearly in a state of deep emotion (possibly allied to feelings of guilt), his hand was suddenly afflicted with *ṣāra'at*, which here too is described as "like snow" (vv. 6–7). Possibly this was simply intended to warn Moses of his sin, for it rapidly disappeared. Allowing for literary licence with regard to the time period involved, this may have represented a brief attack of psoriasis. A longer attack, perhaps again precipitated by emotion, occurred on Mount Sinai, when Moses was alone with God for forty days (Exodus 34:28–35). During this time he was unaware that "the skin of his face glistened," but when he came down it was noticed by the people, who feared to approach him until he had covered his face. Had the shine been due to sunburn, it would not have been painless nor, just as with sweat, would he have needed to put on a mask. This must indicate that the people feared that he suffered from some contagious condition, probably *ṣāra'at* (see below and Leviticus 13:45), although the passage says nothing about it. Since he was not isolated by the priests, it would seem that they recognized the condition as non-contagious and no more than an attack of psoriasis. On the

surely have been aware of her condition. This was particularly the case since, as will be seen, Aaron, as a priest, possessed expert knowledge of such lesions. Aaron then admitted their sin, but his horrified response seems to imply that he was expecting some far more serious retribution for Miriam than a fresh attack of chronic psoriasis. For he then exclaims to Moses (Numbers 12:12): "Let her not become as [a] dead [thing, as one] that comes out from the womb of its mother and its flesh is half eaten away."

In this literal version from the Hebrew, the meaning of the passage is ambiguous. It is usually translated in line with the more picturesque, but no less ambiguous rendering in the Authorized Version of the Bible, whereby Aaron fears that Miriam might become "as one dead, of whom the flesh is half consumed when he cometh out of his mother's womb." Following the Babylonian Talmud (*Avodah zarah* I.1;1a), the phrase "as one dead" is often interpreted without consideration for the rest of the verse. Miriam's "leprous" state is then likened to that of a corpse, which according to Numbers 19:11–14 is to be considered as unclean. It is implied that, due to the shame and distress caused by the inability to play a normal part in society, life is no longer worth living.[33]

In its context, however, the literal translation, "as a dead thing",[34] can only refer to a dead aborted foetus, to which Miriam's physical state is then likened. It is interpreted in this way in the Septuagint, where the description is followed by the words *hosei ektroma*, as in the Vulgate, which gives *ut abortivum*. As any reference to a foetus is absent in the Hebrew text as we have it, these probably represent a gloss. The Septuagint then goes on to say that "half of her (that is, Miriam's) flesh was consumed" (v. 12): in other words, her physical condition is further compared to that of a macerated foetus. Unlike the Hebrew Bible and the Septuagint, the Vulgate also explains that the flesh was "half consumed" due to "lepra". As noted above, in Roman medicine this lat-

---

physical cause of the glistening of psoriatic skin lesions, see L. Fry, *Atlas of Psoriasis* (Carnforth: Parthenon, 1992), 25.

[33]This interpretation does not fit the context of Numbers 12, although it is appropriate for the other Biblical cases quoted in this Talmudic passage, which are taken from quite different contexts: these concern the poor (Proverbs 19:4, 7), the barren (Genesis 30:1, 23), and the blind (Lamentations 3:6).

[34]As in the translations of Luther: *Die Bibel* (Stuttgart: Württembergische Anstalt, 1930); P. Heinisch, *Das Buch Numeri* (Bonn: Hanstein, 1936); and as paraphrased by A. Knobel, *Die Bücher Numeri, Deuteronium und Josua* (Leipzig: Herzel, 1861), 61.

ter term seems to have indicated psoriasis: only in much later times did it come to be applied to true leprosy.[35]

Hence, while initially Miriam only showed signs of chronic psoriasis "like snow", Aaron's reference to "half-consumed" flesh[36] appears to indicate some severe complication of her *ṣāra'at*, during which the reddened skin would peel off in large strips, as with a foetus macerated *in utero*.

Moses was apparently so distressed at Aaron's appraisal that he "cried out to" (or "shouted at", *yitshak*) God to "cure" Miriam (v. 13). While the "curing" or "healing" of various afflictions is repeatedly mentioned in the Bible, here alone is the term applied to a case of *ṣāra'at* that accords with the signs of psoriasis. Only God could actually "cure" a disease, and this may account for the appeal to "cure" (*le-rappe'*) Miriam's condition.[37] Yet even God does not "cure" an incurable disease. Here the term seems to refer not to Miriam's chronic psoriasis, which could be relieved but not cured, but to the threatened onset of an *acute* complication—a far more serious condition. This was doubtless then considered as a separate "disease" that, unlike chronic psoriasis, would not necessarily recur. Thus, if the patient recovered, he was "cured".

Indeed, a condition now known as acute generalized pustular psoriasis occasionally occurs as a dreaded complication of the simple chronic state, and it may even threaten the life of the sufferer. It too can be triggered by psychological factors and toxic reactions, and then lead to severe inflammation with general excoriation of the skin. If secondary infection ensues, the condition becomes truly contagious.[38]

---

[35]Consequently the words "as one dead" have also been widely understood to refer to the attitude to a "leper" that has been customary since medieval times at least. Miriam's "leprous" appearance is then compared to that of a dead foetus, as by C. B. Gray, *Numbers, International Critical Commentary on the Holy Scriptures*, ed. S. R. Driver *et al.* (Edinburgh: Clark, 1903), 127; K. van der Toorn, *Sin and Sanction in Israel and Mesopotamia* (Assen: van Gorcum, 1985), 30–1.

[36]According to Hulse, "The Nature of Biblical 'Leprosy'," 93, 98, this alludes to the tiny bleeding points on the skin, which harmlessly appear when a plaque of simple chronic psoriasis is rubbed off (Auspitz's sign: see Fry, *Atlas of Psoriasis*, 25). The term is interpreted by Lloyd Davies ("Biblical Leprosy," 622) as the desquamation that follows "scarlet fever or other streptococcal infection", once the acute phase is over and the patient is on the way to recovery. However, neither condition would inspire dread; nor would the simile be otherwise apt.

[37]See H. Rouillard, "El rofé en Nombres 12, 13," *Semitica* 37 (1987): 17–46; also n. 45 below.

[38]See H. Baker and T. J. Ryan, "Generalised Pustular Psoriasis," *British Journal of Dermatology*, 80 (1968): 771–93; Mier, *Textbook of Psoriasis*, 9–10; Roenigk, *Psoriasis*, 23–43. In his

If Miriam suffered from chronic psoriasis, she may have recognized premonitory symptoms that such a complication was impending. In any case Aaron, as a priest, should have been fully aware of the existence of this dangerous condition. Thus, his anguished cry, comparing her to a dead "thing", may *additionally* refer to the state of near-death that often occurs in this condition. She was appropriately "shut up outside the camp" for seven days of observation (vv. 14–15),[39] since the condition may take a few days to develop. However, in the event God must have answered the appeals of Aaron and Moses, for she was then allowed to return to the camp, and the people resumed their march through the desert (vv. 15–16). The Bible provides no further information on her state. Perhaps, in her panic before God, Miriam imagined that she felt warnings of this feared complication and raised a false alarm. Alternatively, the condition may have aborted spontaneously.[40] In the event, she apparently suffered no more than an attack of simple chronic psoriasis, for which, as will be seen, isolation was not required.

Whatever its medical interpretation, she was afflicted with *ṣāra'at* for her sin. Yet Aaron went unpunished, although he was equally guilty. Many "common sense" suggestions have been offered to account for this fact but, whatever the cause, it may also reflect those workings of nature that we now call the laws of heredity.[41]

Although, in the cases of Moses and Miriam, attacks of *ṣāra'at* appear to have served as a warning against lack of faith in God, the following "case history", in II Kings 5, seems to indicate that this condition was not always attributed to sin. This is one of three accounts of *ṣāra'at* from a much later period, when the Israelites had for centuries been settled in their land.

---

novel *The Singing Detective* (London: Faber and Faber, 1986) and in his remarkable television film based on this work, the late Dennis Potter, who himself suffered from this dramatic complication of psoriasis, presents a graphic account of its psychological basis and of the physical suffering it engenders.

[39] As noted below, Leviticus 13:4–5 determines the observation period for *ṣāra'at* as seven days, which can once be repeated. This standard number, so often found in ancient instructions of all kinds, represents a suitable median, a guideline for an action that requires about a week.

[40] One might hazard that in the ancient Jewish literary tradition, the latter is implied by a cryptic wordplay on the concept of "abortion", with reference to Numbers 12:12.

[41] Not all members of a family are necessarily affected by a given hereditary disease. It must be noted, moreover, that the actual blood relationship between Moses and Aaron is not entirely clear; see M. D. Rehm, "Levites and Priests," *Anchor Bible Dictionary*, ed. D. N. Freedman (New York: Doubleday, 1992), IV, 298–9.

During the ninth century BC Naaman, an Aramaean army commander honoured even by his Israelite neighbours, had long suffered from *ṣāra'at* (II Kings 5:1). He was advised to consult the Hebrew prophet Elisha although, as noted below, the priests normally dealt with this condition. Elisha recommended that Naaman "bathe seven times in the River Jordan" (v. 10). Having "submerged" himself in this way, "his flesh returned to him like the flesh of a young child and he became clean (*ṭahor*)" (v. 14).

In this description of *ṣāra'at* there is no mention of whiteness, nor is the condition likened to snow. Their absence does not exclude the diagnosis of psoriasis, although it makes it somewhat less certain. Scabies has been often suggested, since it is possible to cure this by bathing.[42] However, the parasitic mite that causes this harmless but truly contagious infestation of the skin is only affected by bathing in hot water with a high sulphur content. Such properties are absent from the Jordan River itself where, according to vv. 10 and 12, Naaman was specifically ordered to bathe. Although they exist in certain "healing" hot springs, no such springs lie on the Jordan or even nearby.[43] Moreover, as will be seen, Naaman's disease was apparently hereditary and scabies would thus be excluded.

This is the only Biblical reference to the actual treatment of *ṣāra'at*. Yet, only a few types of skin lesion are affected by bathing, even in medicinal waters, unless they are secondarily infected. Thorough washing alone would help to heal the chronically infected "desert sores", which so commonly affect soldiers serving under desert conditions; but in such a case scarring is likely to result, rather than entirely "clean" flesh.

However, the uncomplicated skin lesions of chronic psoriasis can uniquely be *relieved* by repeated washing in water. Naaman is instructed to bathe "seven times",[44] which should be sufficient to soften the scaly plaques. These then

---

[42]See Gramberg, " 'Leprosy' and the Bible," 18. According to J. G. Andersen, *Studies in the Mediaeval Diagnosis of Leprosy in Denmark* (Copenhagen: Coster, 1969), 15, scabies would here indicate a "broadening of the purely religious word *ṣāra'at* into a general understanding of uncouthness. . . indicating a person unwanted in the gang." In fact, unless the lesions of scabies are extremely widespread and secondarily infected, the sufferer would hardly be considered as "uncouth".

[43]According to N. Glueck, *The River Jordan* (Philadelphia: Westminster Press, 1946), 46, and also to M. Cogan and H. Tadmor, eds., *Anchor Bible: II Kings* (New York: Doubleday, 1988), 65, Naaman bathed in the hot springs of Hammat Gader, several kilometres east of the River Jordan.

[44]On the significance of bathing "seven" times, see n. 39 above. The action would be enhanced by the running water of any river, but especially by the "jacuzzi" effect of whirlpools

can be easily rubbed off, leaving smooth, pinkish skin, like "that of a child". It was therefore considered as *ṭahor*, "clean" or "pure" (vv. 13–14). Unfortunately, when the lesions of psoriasis are thus removed, the resultant state of "cleanness" is temporary indeed. Yet it is sufficient to send the sufferer home with his condition greatly relieved, and possibly believing himself permanently cured.[45]

The Hebrew term *ṭahor* appears several times in connection with Naaman's *ṣāra'at*, but it is not found in any other "case history", although elsewhere in the Old Testament it is frequently used. It will be noted below that in the priestly code of Leviticus it may also denote spiritually "pure" or "undefiled". However, as Naaman was not Jewish, the question of *ritual* cleanness or purity cannot arise. In this context at least, the term *ṭahor* appears to mean "clean", solely in the physical sense.

The honourable nature of Naaman is continually stressed. As a non-Jew he could hardly be accused of lack of faith in God, and the Bible says nothing of any other sin; nor, uniquely among these "case histories", is his affliction regarded as a punishment.

Perhaps because he was no priest, Elisha refused all remuneration for his aid (vv. 15–16). Later, however, his servant Gehazi secretly approached Naaman, from whom he requested gifts and received them, although denying

---

or eddies, which have been reported in the Jordan a few miles north of the Dead Sea. Traditionally considered as the place where Jesus was baptised, this is where "lepers" are said to have bathed (in the Middle Ages at least) and to have been "cleansed" of their disease. See Gregory of Tours, *In gloria martyrum* xvi; ed. B. Krusch, *Monumenta Germaniae historica, Scriptores rerum merovingicarum,* I.2 (Hanover: Bibliopolus Hahniani, 1884), 499. The bones of leprosy sufferers from about AD 600 have been found in the area; see J. Zias, "Leprosy in the Byzantine Monasteries of the Judean Desert," *Koroth* 9 (1985): 242–7. While lepers may thus have bathed here, this would not preclude its further use to relieve the skin lesions of psoriasis (that is, as a quick "cure"), for which it was certainly more efficacious. Perhaps this was one reason why Naaman was recommended to bathe in the Jordan, rather than in his own Syrian rivers (II Kings 5:12).

[45] Realization of the true nature of the treatment of chronic psoriasis may underlie the fact that here (vv. 3, 6, 7, 10, 11), as throughout the Old Testament, the term *āsaf*—that is, "gather up" rather than "cure"—is used with regard to skin lesions suggestive of this condition, and of this condition alone. Elisha "gathers up" Naaman from his *ṣāra'at*, which seems to indicate that he simply freed the sufferer from his present "attack" of what was recognized as an incurable disease, even though the skin appeared physically "clean". The fact that this term is restricted to such cases, when used in conjunction with disease, may confirm that the condition in question is psoriasis; this conclusion is not abrogated by the one partial exception regarding "cure", noted in Miriam's "case history". See also E. Lieber, " 'Cleansing' the 'Leper' in the Old and New Testaments," *Korot*, in press.

the charge when taxed with it by Elisha (vv. 20–5). The prophet thereupon announced that "the *ṣāra'at* of Naaman" would "stick... forever" to Gehazi and to "his seed". Gehazi then left the presence of his master "afflicted with *ṣāra'at* like snow" (v. 27). Once again psoriasis appears to be indicated, with the initial attack triggered by Gehazi's emotional state.[46] The term *tidbak* is translated as "stick", although in modern Hebrew it would indicate that the condition was contagious. Here, however, it simply appears to denote that it was fitting for Gehazi to be punished with the same disease that afflicted Naaman.

Since all these accounts of *ṣāra'at* are found in Biblical homilies, they may include many similar elements. Yet each contains certain items that vouch for its "medical" authenticity. However, in order to influence the people, such stories must have been based on matters within their experience. Thus, the repeated allusion to one particular condition—apparently chronic psoriasis—tends to show that it was a common scourge in those times and that its features were well known to the public.

As a final example of *ṣāra'at*, the Bible presents the very different case of King Uzziah (Azariah), who reigned from 781–740 BC (II Chronicles 26 and II Kings 15:1–7). The king attempted to usurp a ritual task in the Jerusalem Temple, allotted by God to the priests (II Chronicles 26:16). On being rebuked by the latter, he flew into a rage and "*ṣāra'at* broke out on his forehead" (II Chronicles 26:17–20). He was immediately expelled from the Temple and deposed. He dwelt in a "separate house" (II Chronicles 26:21, II Kings 15:5),[47] and continued to suffer from the condition until the day of his death (II Chronicles 26:21).

---

[46] Gehazi's punishment was also due to lack of faith: in this case not in God, but in his master, the prophet, who served as God's representative. If the remission of Naaman's lesions were expected to be only temporary, it would have been politic for Elisha to let Naaman return home as quickly as possible, without any hindrance from Gehazi. For another suggestion, see van der Toorn, *Sin and Sanction*, 74.

[47] No satisfactory explanation has yet been offered for the Hebrew term used here: *bet hahofshit* (or *hofshut*). On possible interpretations, see Preuss, *Biblical and Talmudic Medicine*, 336; Koehler and Baumgartner, *Lexicon*, I, *s.v. Bet hofshut* or *hofshit*, which seems to indicate a "house of freedom"! Perhaps, as stressed in Leviticus 13:46 (see below), such sufferers were simply ordered to "dwell alone" and thus did not infect other members of their household. As the phrase is explained in the Babylonian Talmud (*Arakhin* IIIv;16b): "He separated a man from his wife, a man from his neighbours." It is clear that, provided that they satisfied the other conditions of the Biblical verse, they were not physically confined to their place of isolation.

This too may have been an attack of psoriasis, which typically appears on the forehead and could have been triggered by the king's outbreak of wrath. Yet this case in particular is often considered as true leprosy, especially as Uzziah was isolated for life. The eruption on the forehead is then thought to indicate a *leonine facies*.[48]

Despite the limited evidence, it seems possible that Uzziah did indeed suffer from leprosy. However, if this be the case, the verse does not refer to such a late manifestation, but to the initial thickening of the skin of the forehead, which may occur relatively early. Rendered more obvious by the king's fit of anger, the condition could then have been recognized by the experienced eyes of the priests, standing immediately before him (II Chronicles 26:19).[49] This identification would certainly account for the fact that Uzziah is treated so harshly, particularly when contrasted with the other cases of *ṣāra'at*, in which psoriasis appears to be indicated.

Thus, in these few Biblical "case histories" the term *ṣāra'at* generally seems to refer to chronic psoriasis, a condition quite harmless to others. However, one case from a late period is here identified as leprosy, indubitably a contagious disease.

Ṣāra'at in law and in ritual

The pericope Numbers 5:1–4 includes what is probably the oldest known version of the actual laws of *ṣāra'at* and the other so-called "purity laws". Here the Israelites, while wandering through the desert, are commanded by God to "send away from the camp" every man or woman suffering from *ṣāra'at*, or from a discharge from the genito-urinary tract, and "everyone who has been made unclean by a dead body", in order that "they should not defile their camps in which I dwell". This brief exhortation thus concentrates on one matter alone: the total isolation of such "unclean" persons from the community, for an unspecified period of time, until they "recovered" or died.

[48] See Muntner, in Rosner, *Medicine in the Bible and Talmud*, 11; M. Stol, "Leprosy: New light from Greek and Babylonian sources," *Ex oriente lux (JEOL)* 30 (1987–8): 22–31. More recent views, however, are typified by Gramberg, " 'Leprosy' and the Bible," 18, who suggests that leprosy would be the most likely identification "on clinical grounds", were it not for the fact that this condition is always described in the Bible "(as white) as snow", and this term is absent in the case of King Uzziah.

[49] Alternatively, early in the course of his leprosy Uzziah's emotional upset may have provoked an acute leprotic reaction, which sometimes occurs within hours. See Canizares, *Clinical Tropical Dermatology*, 188.

The passage can be no more than a summary, thus possibly omitting any references to extenuating circumstances or modifications, such as were included in the much fuller version of these laws found in Leviticus 11–15. Even so, it seems difficult to reconcile these apparently uncompromising commandments with the attitude adopted in the "case histories", particularly the fact that of all these cases of *ṣāra'at*, only King Uzziah was isolated for life. These accounts show little relationship between this affliction and the requirement of exclusion from the "camp". Even the concept of "unclean" is not mentioned, while the term "clean" is used solely with regard to the disease of Naaman, where it seems to signify the actual disappearance of the skin lesions.

On the other hand, it is somewhat surprising that in Numbers 5 neither sin nor punishment are mentioned or even implied, although they feature prominently in the "case histories". But even in the latter *ṣāra'at* was not inflicted as a general punishment for sin, but rather as retribution for some failure in an individual's relationship to God. Moreover, nothing is said of spiritual "uncleanness", or of any form of "atonement".

There is no doubt that the rulings of Numbers 5:2–3 reflect the unique situation of those Israelites who were exiled to the desert after generations of settled life in Egypt. Although quite unused to a nomadic existence, they appear to have rapidly organized their "camp" along military lines—this was the only way to ensure their survival in such an adverse environment. It must necessarily have included measures aimed consciously at controlling the spread of "contagion" by the various communicable diseases, chronic as well as acute, that they encountered on their march through the desert. Initially these would have been adopted from the general experience of desert dwellers, which had gradually evolved over the millennia. Under such circumstances a policy of total exclusion for certain conditions and partial exclusion for others would even be justified today.

The Bible provides few details about acute epidemics, but as will be seen, it deals at length with the management of certain endemic *chronic* conditions encompassed by the cryptic term *ṣāra'at.* Presumably, the latter constituted no less of a hazard to the public, but they required to be dealt with quite differently. Some of these diseases may have been new to the Israelites; but old or new, they required other measures of control that reflected the desert environment. Such control was entrusted to the priests and incorporated into the only legal system of the time, the laws of religion and ritual, for only in this way could the compliance of the people be assured.

Yet unlike the priests of most other religions, those of ancient Israel were in no sense physicians and made no claim whatsoever to be so. In fact, they played little part in the general care of the sick, except to pray for recovery.[50] Acquired mainly from practical experience and camouflaged by the trappings of religion, their measures are not described in medical terms. They are presented in Leviticus 13–14 as legal and ritual rulings, and form part of those chapters of the Bible now known as the "purity laws" (Leviticus 11–15). The remainder deal with animals suitable for food (Leviticus 11), with genito-urinary discharges (Leviticus 15) and with procedures following childbirth (Leviticus 12). In all these very different cases it is repeatedly stressed (as, for example, in Leviticus 11:46–7, 13:59, 14:57) that the primary aim was to distinguish between a person, animal or object that is "unclean" (*tamē'*: "impure", "defiled") and one that is "clean" (*ṭahor*: "pure", "undefiled"); and the "purity laws" consist essentially of the criteria for these terms.

All these laws specify in detail the role of the priests as the sole final arbiters in the recognition of *ṣāra'at* and the other conditions there designated, in the assessment of these cases as "clean" or "unclean", and in their "disposal" (in the military–medical sense), particularly with regard to isolation. Nothing is known about the training of the priests in this field. Yet great expertise and skill were required even for such tasks. For although so restricted in scope, it will be seen that they served to prevent and to limit certain specific chronic infections. However, these roles were so circumscribed and their procedures differed so greatly from those used today that the priests can in no way be compared to modern physicians.[51]

On the other hand, like Numbers 5:2–3, Leviticus 13 makes no mention of sin or its punishment and yet, according to Leviticus 14, in addition to physical "cleansing", "atonement" rituals are required before a person who is deemed to have recovered from *ṣāra'at* can be released from long-term isolation. In some of the "purity laws" the state of "uncleanness" obviously refers to

[50]While the existence of lay "physicians" is occasionally noted in the Bible, God alone is the healer, as in Exodus 15:26: "I, the Lord, [am] thy healer;" Deuteronomy 32:39: "I kill and I make to live; I wound and I heal." However, some prophets, such as Elisha, were apparently delegated by God to "heal", a term that, as noted above, refers not to *ṣāra'at* but to acute "curable" conditions. See D. P. Wright and R. N. Jones, art. "Leprosy" in *Anchor Bible Dictionary*, IV, 278–81: "Prophets heal, priests diagnose." Yet, like many others, Elliger, "Leviticus," 181, somewhat ambivalently considers that the priests "served at the same time as physicians", although their medical "diagnoses" were made primarily for "cultic-religious" purposes.

[51]As they are often considered today, as by Neuberger, "History and Management of AIDS," 34–5.

the person concerned and not to the lesion alone: for example, in the case of a man with a genito-urinary discharge (Leviticus 15:1–15). Similarly, according to Leviticus 14 "purification" is applied to the sufferer as a whole, rather than solely to the lesion. This might seem to justify value judgements regarding the infliction in question. Yet elsewhere in the "purity laws" the text is often ambivalent, while in some cases, as in Leviticus 13:13 and 17, it is the skin manifestations of *ṣāraʿat* that are considered as "clean" or "unclean" and are "purified", hence eliminating any moral connotation. Thus the term *tamē'* in Leviticus appears to refer to a state of physical "uncleanness" that may or may not be accompanied by moral defilement; and the converse applies to *ṭahor*. The physical sense of "unclean" is in no way overruled by the spiritual. This attitude is also expressed in the fragments of an exegesis of Leviticus 13, found in the Dead Sea version of the Damascus Scroll, which dates from around the first century BC. Here *ṣāraʿat* is described not only graphically, as in the Biblical version, but also "in the context of a concrete physiological description".[52]

In the light of modern knowledge it would therefore seem logical to postulate that the fear of physical contagion plays some role in this concept of physical "uncleanness". Yet, partly because of the theological and legal presentation of the "purity laws", there is a general disinclination to interpret them in this way. As has been seen, it is still widely held that all are grounded in ritual alone.[53] The sufferer is thus proclaimed "unclean" or "impure" solely on moral or spiritual criteria.

This theme has been developed in numerous permutations and combinations by Professor Mary Douglas and her school. Thus "the abominations of Leviticus are the obscure unclassifiable elements that do not fit the pattern of

[52]J. M. Baumgarten, "The 4Q Zadokite Fragments on Skin Disease," *Journal of Jewish Studies* 41 (1990): 153–65.

[53]This is not to belittle the positive role of ritual in social affairs, including "public health" matters. Many ancient religions appear to have introduced in this way rational and effective measures for the control of certain prevalent diseases, chronic as well as acute. Despite its relevance to Leviticus 13–14, this problem cannot be adequately discussed here and two examples must suffice. Thus, Pliny (*Natural History* XVIII.7–8) tells of rulings presented to the people in supernatural terms, which were clearly intended for the promotion of health and for the prevention of disease. Again, the early traditions of Islam include instructions for the prevention of contagion. People living in a plague-stricken area should not flee elsewhere, but such a place should be avoided by those unaffected by the condition; see L. I. Conrad, "Epidemic Disease in Formal and Popular Thought in Early Islamic Society," in T. Ranger and P. Slack, eds., *Epidemics and Ideas* (Cambridge: Cambridge University Press, 1992), 97–8.

the cosmos. They are incompatible with holiness and blessing."[54] Although referring to Leviticus 21:17–23, the citation exemplifies this attitude towards Leviticus 13 and the other "purity laws". The consequent state of "impurity" or "pollution" then represents the priestly stick that ensures the compliance of the people. "Impurity" is no euphemism for physical "contagion". It is a purely ritual concept, which on no account should be taken at face value, and its ultimate "danger" lies in social and physical ostracism.[55]

The dangerous "pollution" specified in the "purity laws" is thus ascribed to taxonomic or other anomalies of persons, animals or objects. Yet, when applied, for example, to the "forbidden" foods of Leviticus 11:26,[56] this hardly explains why an animal that does not chew the cud or possess cloven hooves, such as the pig, should be considered "abnormal"—let alone a danger to society—compared, for example, to a cow.

"Medical" explanations of such social or anthropological phenomena are dismissed as aspects of "medical (or scientific) materialism", using this term in a purely pejorative sense.[57] Any "medical" advantage accruing from the "purity laws" is then solely regarded as a "side-benefit".[58]

Even this brief introduction demonstrates the inadequacy of any interpretation of the "purity laws" that ignores their "medical" connotations. In fact, in this study the standpoint of "medical materialism"—albeit in a positive sense—has been intentionally adopted as an aid to understanding the Biblical concept of *ṣāra'at*.

---

[54] M. Douglas, *Purity and Danger* (London: Routledge, 1966), 95.

[55] Ibid., 32. For a typical theological adoption of these theories, see G. J. Wenham, "The Book of Leviticus" in *New International Commentary on the Old Testament*, ed. R. K. Harrison (London: Hodder and Stoughton, 1979), 192: the manifestations of "impurity" decreed in the "purity laws" (such as skin lesions or bodily discharges) are considered as clearly "abnormal and by disfiguring the appearance of man and his works destroy the wholeness that ought to characterize the creation. For this reason such conditions are pronounced as unclean." Yet, see *Leviticus, The Pentateuch and Haftorahs*, ed. J. H. Hertz (London: Oxford University Press, 1932), for the acceptance by an orthodox Jewish theologian of a role for contagion in the "purity laws" as a whole, especially the brief but inspired introduction (110–11) and observations on dietary laws (94), childbirth (111–12), and physical secretions (144).

[56] M. Douglas, "Deciphering a Meal", in her *Implicit Meanings* (London: Routledge and Kegan Paul, 1975), 266–306.

[57] Douglas, *Purity and Danger*, 32. Such usage of the term "medical materialism" has been adapted from its original application by W. James, *The Varieties of Religious Experience* (London: Longman's, 1907), 13, to those who dismiss the concept of "religious states of mind", because these may be due to some pathological lesion of the body.

[58] Douglas, *Purity and Danger*, 29. See also n. 23 above.

The rulings of Leviticus 13–14 on the question of *ṣāraʿat* represent a long development of legal practice, beginning with the time of the expulsion from Egypt and the subsequent wandering in the desert, as glimpsed in Deuteronomy 24:8–9.[59] Based partly on records from the Jerusalem Temple, they go on to reflect the later centuries when the Israelites led a settled existence in their land under totally different social and environmental conditions. In their Masoretic form these prescriptions were then "edited" during the upheavals of the Babylonian exile and the subsequent return to the homeland in the sixth to fifth centuries BC. However, since all this is highly compressed in our texts, it is difficult to distinguish between the changes and modifications of the rulings at different periods of time, or to determine their chronological order.

The conflation is partly masked by the uniform presentation of the rules of *ṣāraʿat*. As with all the "purity laws", the investigations legally prescribed in order to distinguish the "clean" from the "unclean" are essentially arranged according to a binary ("yes–no") system, as shown in the table below with regard to Leviticus 13. They are set out in the form of protasis–apodosis, whereby the observation stipulated ("if. . . ") is followed by a resultant prognosis ("then. . . "). This was the traditional form of the Near Eastern omen texts (primarily from Mesopotamia), particularly of those based on hepatoscopy, which had long been employed in divination.[60] Here, as in Leviticus 13, the prognosis was based entirely on visual indications. Such a standardized system required only the minimum of training and thus could be administered by priests who lacked any medical expertise.

According to the ritual laid down in Leviticus 13, any person suffering from certain specified skin lesions "resembling a *negaʿ ṣāraʿat*" had to be brought before a priest (v. 2). The term *negaʿ* is not found in the "case histories". From its derivation it indicates something acquired by contact: by a touch, or by a blow—originally, perhaps, "seizure" by a demon.[61] Hence, in the Bible it came to denote a misfortune inflicted by God, such as an "attack" of a disease,

---

[59] Elliger, "Leviticus," 179–80. The Bible also provides other evidence of these priestly rules in pre-exilic times, as in Deuteronomy 24:8–9.

[60] See I. Starr, *The Rituals of the Diviner* (Malibu: Undena, 1983), *passim*; E. Lieber, " 'He Looked in the Liver' (Ezekiel 21:26): the Medical Origins of Liver Divination," *Koroth* 9 (1988): 235–45.

[61] Perhaps "seizure" by a disease-bearing demon; see Elliger, "Leviticus," 180. On this concept of disease in ancient Mesopotamia, see J. Black and A. Green, *Gods, Demons and Symbols of Ancient Mesopotamia* (London: British Museum Press, 1992), 67.

an "affliction", a "lesion", or, as in the Authorized Version of Exodus 11:1, a "plague" (from the Latin *plaga*: a "blow", as in the Vulgate), in the sense of some terrible blow or misfortune.

The very early concept of seizure by a demon might already seem to indicate "contagion". Yet in Leviticus 13–14 *nega'* does not appear to be used in this sense, even though, as will be seen, it is usually linked there with *ṣāra'at* and it is repeatedly hinted that some types of *ṣāra'at* are contagious.[62] Hence, the term *nega' ṣāra'at* simply constituted a legal formula, used to proclaim that the condition in question indubitably represented an "attack" or "affliction" of *ṣāra'at*, although not necessarily in the purely physical sense of a "lesion".[63]

The suspected case of *ṣāra'at* was probably examined in the presence of a witness, the person who had "brought" him to the priest. No practical steps could be taken until the priest had formally proclaimed that the condition of *ṣāra'at* was present and that it was "clean" or "unclean". In cases of difficulty the sufferer could be "shut up" for observation, for two separate seven-day periods (v. 5).[64]

This principle of categorizing *ṣāra'at* itself as "unclean" or "clean" was unique among the "purity laws" and constituted a major deviation from the rigid stipulations of Numbers 5:2–3. If it was proclaimed as "unclean", the sufferer was required "to live alone, outside the camp" (v. 46), until recovery or death supervened. However, as will be seen, a "clean" case of *ṣāra'at* was only potentially contagious. Thus, such a sufferer was apparently excluded only from the Sanctuary or Temple, being thereby prevented from making the mandatory sacrifices.[65]

All decisions regarding release from these conditions were also the prerogative of the priest, who first proclaimed the sufferer as "clean" on physical grounds and then performed the rituals of "purification" or "cleansing", as described in Leviticus 14:1–32. In any dispute on the matter, it was he who had the last word (Deuteronomy 21:5). Most important of all, he alone could ensure the enforcement of the law, including the matter of isolation. Thus, even from the purely medical aspect, the priests wielded great power.

---

[62] Hence Preuss, *Biblical and Talmudic Medicine*, 326: "*Nega*, in and of itself is a general concept: contagion."

[63] See Sawyer, "A Note on the Etymology of *Ṣāra'at*," 241–5.

[64] On the significance of the duration of this period, see n. 39 above.

[65] See Hertz, *Leviticus*, 111, 115.

Ṣāraʿat as a medical concept in law

Unlike the "case histories" presented above, the rules of Leviticus 13:1–46 and 14:1–32 are designed to assess, from the legal point of view, whether *ṣāraʿat* is present and whether it is "clean" or "unclean". Even when humans are affected, no value judgements are involved. The criteria consist only of physical signs in the skin: all easily visible to the sufferer, the priest, and probably to a witness as well.

Leviticus 13:1–46 is customarily divided into an introductory verse and six sections, consisting of vv. 2–8, 9–17, 18–23, 24–8, 29–37 and 38–46. These roughly follow a general pattern: first an "index lesion" or "clear case" is presented, and this is followed by a number of variants exemplifying problematic cases that may be found difficult to categorize.[66]

Verse 2 designates three types of lesion as "resembling a *negaʿ ṣāraʿat*": *seʾet*, *sappahat* and *baheret*; but it is possible that only the first was originally specified.[67] Whatever the ruling, it seems to show that the public possessed some idea of the kind of lesions involved: no doubt from priestly instruction (see Deuteronomy 24:8 and Ezekiel 44:23). However, the Bible provides no definitions or descriptions of these terms and, despite numerous modern suggestions, their interpretation still remains unclear. The translations offered by the Authorized Version—a "rising", a "scab" and a "bright spot"—are in general as plausible as any, although in certain contexts these terms might also indicate, respectively, a "swelling", a "scaly patch" or a "scab" and a "light" or "shiny" spot.

If in any of the above "index lesions" the hair in the lesion has turned white and the lesion itself appears to be lower than the skin, the case is to be proclaimed as a *negaʿ ṣāraʿat* and is to be considered as "unclean". Additionally, as in v. 4 and elsewhere, the white appearance of the lesion may serve to confirm the condition. While these are the essential *positive* criteria that confirm the status of the case, rulings in subsequent verses clearly indicate that it may sometimes be decided in the absence of one or more of these signs.

Leviticus 13 then goes on to present further examples of this kind, in order to help the priest to deduce the presence or absence of *ṣāraʿat* and then to

---

[66] For a verse-by-verse analysis, see M. Jastrow Jr., "The So-Called 'Leprosy' Laws," *Jewish Quarterly Review*, New Series, 4 (1914): 357–418; Elliger, "Leviticus," 180–9; J. Wilkinson, "Leprosy and Leviticus," *Scottish Journal of Theology* 30 (1977): 153–69; Seidl, *Tora für den "Aussatz"-Fall*, *passim*.

[67] Elliger, "Leviticus," 168.

distinguish between the "clean" and the "unclean" condition. Thus, while the legal formulation of *nega' ṣāra'at* represents a truly medical *concept,* it was in no way considered at the time as denoting a specific "disease" or "diseases", and the chapter itself provides no interpretation of this kind.

On the other hand, it is now possible to utilize these signs as in medicine today, and obtain a "diagnosis" by induction. When they have been interpreted in this way, it has widely and rightly been noted that the hair is not turned white in the lesions of leprosy, nor even in those of psoriasis; but it is also asserted that, apart from a few rare diseases, this only occurs in vitiligo. As has been seen, vitiligo is a completely innocuous condition, and could hardly bear the burden of *ṣāra'at.* Moreover, while the ruling that the lesion must be lower than the skin clearly denotes ulceration, this sign is entirely non-specific. It is certainly a feature of leprosy, but it also occurs in numerous other conditions, some of which are relatively mild, although it is not found in chronic psoriasis or vitiligo. Hence, as has been seen, it is now generally considered that the concept of *ṣāra'at* does not refer to true leprosy, and many go further and assert that even its *positive* criteria cannot be validated in the light of modern medical knowledge.

However, the enormous literature on Biblical "leprosy" has almost entirely ignored the possibility that during the Exodus the Israelites encountered a highly contagious chronic disease of the desert, of which, even today, little is known in the West. This is bejel (treponarid, endemic syphilis),[68] a non-venereal treponematosis caused by an organism possibly identical with that of syphilis and very similar to that of yaws. The name endemic syphilis is misleading, since bejel is rarely if ever sexually transmitted; but it spreads even more rapidly, by actual contact with highly infectious lesions of the skin or the mouth, particularly by kissing and by the use of common vessels for drinking. In many other respects it must be distinguished from both syphilis and yaws, for since each of these diseases flourishes under different social and environmental conditions, their manifestations too are quite different.

[68] See E. H. Hudson, *Non-Venereal Syphilis* (Edinburgh: Livingstone, 1958), *passim.* The author, one of the few Western physicians with wide clinical experience of bejel among Middle Eastern nomads, also suggests (16, 116) that the condition might represent Biblical "leprosy". However, this possibility does not yet seem to have been considered by Biblical scholars. For purely clinical aspects, see G. W. Csonka, "Clinical Aspects of Bejel," *British Journal of Venereal Diseases* 29 (1953): 95–103; T. J. Ryan, *Microvascular Injury* (London: Saunders, 1976), 200–1; *Manson's Tropical Diseases,* ed. P. E. L. Manson-Bahr and D. R. Bell, 19th ed. (London: Cassell, 1987), 624–6, 639–41; A. Basset and J. Maleville in Canizares, *Clinical Tropical Dermatology,* 143–50.

Bejel occurs in hot dry environments and is generally linked with poor hygiene. It has probably existed for thousands of years in parts of the eastern Mediterranean and Africa,[69] where it is still common today among the desert nomads and villagers, but rarely appears in the towns. Under the particular environmental and social conditions of the Exodus, it could have constituted no less of a danger to the Israelites than acute epidemic conditions, such as smallpox or plague. Sudden contact with a disease of this kind, to which they possessed no immunity, might have threatened their very existence.

This disease is far more contagious than leprosy, to which it bears no relationship at all. It alone produces branny scales on the skin, but both conditions may give rise to whitish depigmentation and deep ulceration of the lesions, which go on to form scars. The late manifestations of bejel are often no less fearful than those of syphilis or leprosy. It too may result in deformities of the limbs and terrible mutilations of the face, including destruction of the nose (*gangosa*), although the sufferers do not exhibit the *leonine facies*, which is distinctive of leprosy alone. Moreover, unlike syphilis and leprosy,

[69] On the history of the treponemal diseases, see Grmek, *Diseases in the Ancient Greek World*, 133–44. He rightly notes that although no human remains bearing sure signs of any treponematosis have been found from before AD 1500, this does not invalidate the theory that such conditions may have existed far earlier. According to R. T. Steinbock, *Paleopathological Diagnosis and Interpretation* (Springfield: Thomas, 1976), 138–9, bone lesions are rare in bejel, so that even in an endemic area, the condition could only be diagnosed "in roughly 1–5 % of the entire series". However, Grmek (142) categorically denies that "the Greek world" knew of bejel, or any other form of treponematosis. Yet, around the turn of the sixth century BC, Aeschylus described in his *Choephori* 277–81 a terrible disease known as *leichēn*, which "ate into the flesh" and whitened the hair. This is considered by Grmek as "a mythic disease" but, according to such commentators as J. Conington, trans., *The Choephoroe of Aeschylus* (London: Parker, 1857), 46; A. F. Garvie (Oxford: Clarendon Press, 1986), 115, it corresponds to Biblical "leprosy", which gave rise to white hair, and thus indicates true leprosy. However, like many cases of Biblical "leprosy", it is probable that this too was bejel. Aeschylus lived at the time when Leviticus 13 was composed; but if the identification with bejel is correct, the condition might already have been present in the eastern Mediterranean for centuries. In his account of skin diseases, over five centuries later (*De medicina* V.28), the Latin author Celsus, who probably knew nothing of bejel, does not mention *leichēn*. However, he seems to have confused the concept of *leichēn* expressed by Aeschylus, with a banal skin condition that he calls *leuke* (ibid. 19A–B). In his description of the latter he modifies the fearful signs of *leichēn* but notes that *leuke* also whitens the hair; he thus rightly classifies it as "a form of vitiligo". Subsequently, Pliny described *leichēn* itself as a "new disease" in Rome—a disfiguring disease with "branny" scales, which he attributes to kissing (*Historia naturalis* XXVI.1–4). This was surely some form of bejel, possibly brought back by Roman soldiers after some desert campaign and resulting in a temporary urban epidemic.

bejel tends to become latent and sometimes spontaneously remits or "burns out".

However, of the greatest importance for our understanding of *ṣāraʿat* is the fact that as in bejel, but not leprosy, the hair tends to turn white[70] and "moth-eaten" patches of baldness typically appear on the scalp. Whitening of the hair is not a feature of any other *serious* endemic condition, and in the relatively banal vitiligo it is not linked with alopecia.

Even so, in the Middle East bejel has long been confused with other chronic endemic conditions, particularly with cutaneous leishmaniasis and leprosy,[71] and later, also with syphilis and yaws.

Cutaneous leishmaniasis[72] has long been prevalent in Mesopotamia. It may first have been encountered by the Israelites in the Jordan valley during the Exodus from Egypt and then, centuries later, during the Babylonian Exile. It usually takes the form of an itching "boil" on the face, covered with fine whitish scales. In most cases this eventually disappears on its own, leaving a scar that remains throughout life. However, the condition may spread, particularly in those who have had little former contact with the disease. This diffuse cutaneous type may give rise to psoriasis-like skin lesions, and it can also produce gross mutilations of the face. Yet, in contrast to bejel and leprosy, none of the lesions are contagious, although they may well have been considered as such, since the condition is highly infectious, being spread by sandflies and rodents. A most important aid in the *early* differentiation of leishmaniasis from bejel is the fact that the former does not whiten the hair.

Hence, in the context of the wandering through the desert, a case of *ṣāraʿat* displaying ulcerated skin lesions and "baldness" (Leviticus 13:42), but in which any hair present has turned white, and for which sometimes there is hope of a "cure" (Leviticus 14:3), seems likely to indicate no other condition than bejel. However, since the skin lesions may be confused with those of other contagious or infectious diseases, as well as with non-contagious psoriasis, a period of observation may be required to confirm the condition. Isolation for only a few weeks (vv. 4–5, see n. 39) would not suffice to differentiate

[70] See Hudson, *Non-Venereal Syphilis*, 116. However, Hulse, "The Nature of Biblical 'Leprosy'," 98, suggests that Leviticus 13 refers to the hair being flecked with the white scales of psoriasis.

[71] In the Middle East both bejel and leprosy are still considered as "unclean"; see Hudson, *Non-Venereal Syphilis*, 17.

[72] On leishmaniasis see Ridley, *Pathogenesis of Leprosy*, 18; Manson-Bahr, *Manson's Tropical Diseases*, 729–73.

leprosy from psoriasis, but would be adequate to distinguish the latter from bejel or cutaneous leishmaniasis.

Yet, although in Leviticus 13 the concept of *ṣāraʿat* thus seems to be targeted primarily at bejel, a fearsome and contagious disease, in the "case histories" it refers mainly to psoriasis (although possibly also to one case of leprosy). This paradox is, however, resolved when vv. 1–46 are analysed as a whole, with the aid of modern medical concepts.

The "clear case" of *ṣāraʿat* in v. 3, which seems to indicate the skin lesions of bejel, is contrasted with a doubtful case in vv. 4–6, in which a white lesion tends to darken but is not deeper than the skin and does not display any white hair. This is clearly not bejel, and if, after two weeks of observation, it "darkens" but does not spread, it is not considered as *ṣāraʿat.* It is only a "scab" and, after washing his clothes, the sufferer is proclaimed to be "clean". Such a "scab" may even represent a self-limiting case of cutaneous leishmaniasis. However, if later the "scab" begins to spread (vv. 7–8), this denotes a more serious condition, perhaps the diffuse psoriatic form of leishmaniasis, which is highly infectious. This is considered as both *ṣāraʿat* and "unclean".

The next "clear case" (vv. 9–11) is represented by an "old" (or chronic) *negaʿ ṣāraʿat,* which had earlier been recognized as such. It had then been proclaimed as "unclean", but when a change occurred in the lesion, it had to be examined anew. A white "rising" had appeared in the skin, within which the hair had turned white and "living" (*ḥay,* perhaps "wild") flesh was exposed. An old skin lesion of bejel had apparently begun to ulcerate. There was no need to "shut up" the sufferer for observation, since he had long been assessed as "unclean".[73]

According to vv. 12–17, if *ṣāraʿat* covers all the body and is white, it is to be considered as "clean". This seems to refer to simple chronic psoriasis, since nothing is said of white hair. However, if "living flesh" appears in the lesion, the *ṣāraʿat* is then rendered "unclean". The change may be due to that dreaded complication of psoriasis, the generalized pustular state, which was suggested above in connection with Miriam's *ṣāraʿat.* If the skin then reverts to its former white state, the *negaʿ* is once again "clean"; this is again only simple psoriasis.

The cases presented in vv. 3–17 epitomize the concept of "clean" and "unclean" *ṣāraʿat* expounded in Leviticus 13 and constitute the model for the remainder of these rules.[74] According to the analysis so far, only skin lesions

[73]See Hertz, *Leviticus,* 118 note to v. 11.

[74]See Jastrow, "The So-Called 'Leprosy' Laws," 360–5.

evocative of a highly contagious chronic disease such as bejel, or the infectious cutaneous leishmaniasis (which was probably thought to be contagious), are proclaimed as both *ṣāra'at* and "unclean". As long as they persist the sufferer must be isolated (as described in vv. 45–6). These lesions are then contrasted with the skin indications of certain chronic but non-contagious conditions with which they can easily be confused, in particular with chronic psoriasis. Although also considered as *ṣāra'at*, such conditions are held to be "clean" and are not totally isolated. However, if serious complications ensue, they are proclaimed as "unclean" and undergo strict isolation until the condition remits.

Vv. 18–23 repeat the pattern of vv. 4–8, but refer now to the changes that may arise in the scar of a healed "boil". The lesion described in vv. 19–20, which displays white hair, is considered as "unclean" and a *nega' ṣāra'at*. It again seems to indicate bejel. This is then contrasted in vv. 22–3 with the same kind of scar, but here white hair or ulceration are absent. If it darkens and then spreads, it is held to be "unclean" and a *nega'* (v. 22). Again, this is possibly diffuse leishmaniasis, spreading from the typical "boil". However, if it darkens without spreading, it is "clean"; it is only the "scar" of the (usually self-limiting) "boil" (v. 23).

The following section (vv. 24–8) deals with the changes that may result in the burn or scar when the "actual cautery", the branding iron (*mikvat esh*), is applied to a "boil" (as is still the practice in the Middle East[75]). This passage too seems to distinguish between the skin lesions of bejel (vv. 24–5) and those of cutaneous leishmaniasis (vv. 26–8).

Vv. 29–37 are concerned with other chronic, but far less serious skin lesions. Again, those proclaimed as *ṣāra'at* and "unclean" appear to be contagious conditions and would thus have to be distinguished from the rest. For example, vv. 29–30 may refer to favus, a fungal infestation of the scalp, or else to some bacterial infection of the hair. In either case, the roots of the hair become surrounded by yellow crusts.

The final section on human *ṣāra'at* (vv. 38–46) deals with the whiteness of the lesions and the type of baldness involved, in order to differentiate between banal "clean" cases and those proclaimed as "utterly unclean". It ends with a graphic description of the "disposal" of the latter (vv. 42–6), which, as suggested above, applied originally to cases of bejel. The conditions of the march through the desert would justify a decree that such a sufferer must "dwell alone (*badad*), outside the camp", as long as the condition persisted

[75] See Hudson, *Non-Venereal Syphilis*, Fig. 4.

(see n. 47). With his "clothes rent and hair unkempt" (that is, uncovered), his skin lesions would be visible to all. His "upper lip" was to be covered by a mask, which would have helped to prevent dissemination of bejel from the highly contagious lesions in the mouth.[76]

It is likely, however, that bejel ceased be a "public health" problem for the Israelites once they were settled in Canaan. Here true leprosy may, to some extent, have taken its place, perhaps even affecting King Uzziah, whose lesions correspond with those described in Leviticus 13:43. Thus, while vv. 42–6 seem originally have been formulated against bejel, they may later have been modified to be also compatible with leprosy, hence omitting any reference to white hair. V. 43 describes typical signs of early leprosy: a reddish-white lesion of the forehead, as well as frontal baldness (possibly including loss of eyebrows), which contrasts with the alopecia of bejel. In this post-exodic conflation the reference to the "camp", although no longer valid, supplied an antique patina for new rulings. It is no wonder, therefore, that our late version of these laws appears ambivalent as well as ambiguous.

The absence of literary evidence and the fact that there exists no palaeopathological evidence of true leprosy in Egypt prior to the second century BC are not decisive criteria, but they have helped to sustain the prevailing idea that leprosy was not present in the Middle East or Egypt before the fourth century BC. It is thus generally thought to have been brought there by Alexander the Great on returning from his Indian campaign.[77]

According to Josephus, who lived in the first century AD, earlier Greek historians, such as Manetho, had claimed that the Jews were exiled from Egypt because Moses among others suffered from *lepra* and other "scabby" conditions, which they then transmitted to others.[78] Here too the term *lepra* has generally been translated as "leprosy". It has, however, been seen that the term is applied to various non-contagious skin conditions—above all to psoriasis, the disease probably inflicted on Moses. Due to its marked hereditary ele-

[76] As regards the rent clothes, still today the clothes of mourners who have been in contact with the dead are symbolically torn at Jewish funerals. No doubt they were once rightly considered as potentially contagious. Elliger, "Leviticus," 185, maintains that although the text only requires the "moustache" to be covered, the ruling must also have included the nose, since this would have protected other people from the entry of disease-bearing spirits through the body's main portal, the respiratory tract.

[77] See Andersen, *Studies*, 45.

[78] *Josephus*, Loeb trans. by H. St. J. Thackeray (London: Heinemann, 1961): *Against Apion* I.279–320; *idem.*, *Jewish Antiquities* III.265–8. See also S. S. Kottek, *Medicine... in the Works of Flavius Josephus* (Leiden: E. J. Brill, 1994), 42–4.

ment, psoriasis may have affected the Jews more than the rest of the population in Egypt. Even so, true leprosy could first have become prevalent in Egypt around the time of the Exodus, in the thirteenth century BC. Although the Jews were not necessarily affected as yet, they might well have been blamed for its spread, by confusion with their chronic psoriasis.

This latter suggestion is based on the finding that a gradual change occurred in the innumerable representations of the popular Egyptian deity Bes. By the period of the Exodus he had come to be generally depicted as a man with a *leonine facies* and other manifestations characteristic only of leprosy.[79] Moreover, this disease continued to be accurately represented for so long that its depiction must have been continually reinforced by the actual observation of such cases. Leprosy in Egypt may well have originated in black Africa, but an Egyptian deity would hardly have been so widely portrayed in this manner had it not been common in Egypt, perhaps occurring at first among resident blacks, but then soon spreading to the indigenous population. Yet with one important exception, the numerous icons of Bes have not been considered as representations of leprosy, nor of any other disease. Although art historians have long noted what they too call a *leonine facies*, this has always been considered as no more than an "artistic convention" for the representation of a leonine deity.

However, a head of Bes on an anthropomorphic clay vessel, dating from around 1300 BC, has been found in an Egyptian temple in Canaan, and it has been claimed that its *leonine facies* shows signs of advanced lepromatous leprosy.[80] When contrasted with an actual case of the condition, manifestations such as the peculiar "frown", due to superciliary infiltration, and the characteristic lagophthalmos, are so accurately depicted that it must have been

[79] See E. Lieber, "Leprosy in the Lands of the Bible, and the Demons Bes and Pazuzu," Part I: "Ancient Egypt and the Bes-Image," *Korot* 10 (1993–4): 25–43.

[80] As first suggested by M. Yoeli, "A *facies leontina* of Leprosy on an Ancient Canaanite Jar," *Journal of the History of Medicine* 10 (1955): 331–5; *idem*, "Mot, the Canaanite God, Symbol of the Leper," *Bulletin of the New York Academy of Medicine* 44 (1968): 1057–67; and supported by Cochrane and Davey, *Leprosy in Theory and Practice*, 1–2. Yet this identification has been widely opposed, as by Hulse, "The Nature of Biblical 'Leprosy'," 87, mainly on the grounds that leprosy did not exist in Egypt at that time. On the earliest evidence of leprosy in Egypt, see Grmek, *Diseases in the Ancient Greek World*, 154, 159. According to Andersen, *Studies*, 16, such a figure would be a curious choice for a jug, unless designated for ritual or magical purposes. However, the presence of the deity may denote that the jug was reserved for the use of such sufferers, due to fear of contagion, and it perhaps served as a warning to the public not to share the use of vessels for drinking or eating. This does not necessarily indicate the confusion of bejel with leprosy, in view of the highly contagious nasal secretions in leprosy.

modelled on actual observation of true leprosy and not merely copied from elsewhere. Thus it can also be clearly distinguished from a representation of bejel, or of diffuse cutaneous leishmaniasis.

Yet this vessel was not necessarily imported from Egypt: it could have been produced in Canaan. This would support an alternative hypothesis: that the Jews first acquired leprosy in Canaan, where it had been brought perhaps from Mesopotamia, at a time when it was still absent from Egypt.[81] On the other hand, it might also have spread there from Egypt. In any case, this is a moot point for the Israelites, since during their wanderings in the desert bejel appears to have constituted a far greater hazard than leprosy.

It has been seen that Leviticus 13 deals solely with the natural course of *ṣāra'at*: sin is neither mentioned nor implied. However, moral considerations are not ignored in these rules, but are concentrated in the following chapter. Yet Leviticus 14:1–32 does not overtly consider even "moral contagion". Here one finds description of atonements and sacrifices that must be performed once physical recovery is confirmed. But the sins for which the *ṣāra'at* was presumably inflicted, and for which "purification" is required, are not specified. Yet, in the "case histories" above, *ṣāra'at* is largely attributed to a particular sin, while atonement is only mentioned with regard to Miriam's affliction (see Numbers 12:11) and, in a more logical sequence, this is said to precede her recovery. This paradox may be partly resolved if Leviticus 14 in its turn is considered as an amalgam of texts old and new. This chapter seems to hint that the ritual washings for "purification" had *also* served as a test to differentiate bejel from psoriasis, while the other materials specified for "cleansing" (as in v. 4) may originally have signified substances for alleviating or healing the lesions.[82] Indications of rational therapy appear to have been later overlaid

[81]Cochrane and Davey, *Leprosy in Theory and Practice*, 1–2; Grmek, *Diseases in the Ancient Greek World*, 162. The latter (159–60) also tends to agree with Kinnear Wilson, "Leprosy in Ancient Mesopotamia," 49–51, that leprosy is described in a Babylonian omen-text of the second millennium BC. Yet the mere mention there of "white patches" and of "dots", whereby the sufferer is rejected by his god and by mankind, is surely insufficient to indicate "the two main types of leprosy," or any other specific disease. Even in combination they might equally represent bejel or cutaneous leishmaniasis.

[82]A test for psoriasis, by washing off the lesions and observing Auspitz's sign, seems to be implied in a Dead Sea fragment from around the first century BC and in a Roman medical work from around the same period; see n. 36 above and E. Lieber, "Chronic Skin Diseases in Ancient Times," paper in preparation. On hints of the treatment of *ṣāra'at* in Leviticus 14, see Jastrow, "The So-Called 'Leprosy' Laws," 369–72, esp. n. 42; Michman, "Leprosy," col. 33; Lieber, "Chronic Skin Diseases in Ancient Times."

(but not cancelled) by ideas of "spiritual cleansing", on a supernatural basis.

Thus, in the concept of *ṣāraʿat* expressed in these chapters of Leviticus, religion and medicine appear to remain independent. Yet in fact they have been carefully dovetailed, in order to complement each other.

Conclusions

It has been suggested above that in the Biblical "case histories" of *ṣāraʿat*, this term refers to chronic psoriasis, a common non-contagious condition, except for one case in which leprosy is possibly indicated. On the other hand, the laws of human *ṣāraʿat*, as summarized in Leviticus 13:1–46 and 14:1–32, are essentially directed at certain specific highly contagious diseases. Neither conclusion accords with the widespread opinion that Leviticus 13 represents diagnostic flow charts "in which certain physical manifestations, not the underlying disease, were signs to the priests to rule whether or not a person was ritually unclean".[83] In fact, the term "unclean" is considered in this paper as referring to a state of physical (and spiritual) "contagion" that may be either actual or potential.

According to Leviticus 13, the main indication of "unclean" *ṣāraʿat* is a skin lesion that ulcerates and in which the hair has turned white. These actually constitute the *early* signs of bejel, and are pathognomonic of bejel alone. This highly contagious, chronic mutilating disease is endemic to Near Eastern deserts. If it were first acquired by the Israelites in the course of the Exodus from Egypt, under the marginal conditions of the desert, it could have threatened their very existence. Other skin signs of "unclean" *ṣāraʿat* may represent the early signs of cutaneous leishmaniasis, a chronic endemic disease that is highly infectious and was probably thought to be contagious. Although nowadays usually mild, it can produce very severe manifestations. It may well have affected the Israelites for a short period during the Exodus, as well as centuries later, during the Babylonian Exile. Moreover, Leviticus 13 may also cover the skin signs of leprosy, a contagious disease that could have replaced bejel as an epidemiological hazard once the Israelites were settled in Canaan.

Thus, from the beginning of the Exodus from Egypt, new and special measures had to be instituted to prevent and contain such chronic "contagious" conditions. To be effective they would essentially depend on the accurate identification of cases, at the earliest possible stage. However, being unused

[83] Wilkinson, "Leprosy and Leviticus," 164–5.

to the diseases that threaten a nomadic existence, the Israelites must have adopted the age-old practices of the desert, based on the principle of "better safe than sorry". It is this type of system that appears to be summarized in Numbers 5:2–4, while the later modifications are conflated in Leviticus 13.

This task of control, based purely on medical criteria, was entrusted solely to the priests, although they were in no way physicians. For they alone could ensure total compliance with the rules, through moral and spiritual pressure. Hence Leviticus 13–14 are couched in terms of law and ritual alone.

As described in Leviticus 13, the assessment was based on visible skin signs or markers, which would be clearly apparent to all. This was possible since, by sheer chance, in all three diseases noted above, the early signs appear in the skin and serve to herald their onset. Thus, on the basis of skin signs alone, the priests could effectively identify a *nega' ṣāra'at* (an "attack" of *ṣāra'at*) at a very early stage of the disease.

From the Old Testament "case histories" of *ṣāra'at*, it appears that non-contagious chronic psoriasis, and perhaps also contagious true leprosy, could serve as punishment for lack of faith in God. On the other hand, Leviticus 13 makes no mention whatsoever of sin, but it too repeatedly describes as *ṣāra'at* skin lesions characteristic of psoriasis, as well as those of highly contagious chronic conditions such as bejel. In the absence of modern treatment it was perfectly rational (and medically effective) to consider the latter as "absolutely unclean", in the sense of physically contagious, and to isolate them strictly and indefinitely (Leviticus 13:45–6).

Yet, as has been seen, the early skin signs of bejel, cutaneous leishmaniasis and leprosy can easily be confused with the skin lesions of chronic psoriasis. Thus, highly contagious diseases might occasionally slip through the net, while some harmless skin lesions could be wrongly assessed as contagious. The latter too would then be condemned to the restrictions of Leviticus 13:46, including isolation until recovery or death supervened.

It is suggested that both types of lesion were therefore deliberately considered as *ṣāra'at*, but were then differentiated as "unclean" and "clean". Those forms assessed as "unclean" appear to correspond with conditions held to be physically contagious. However, lesions that normally constitute no danger to the public, were considered as "clean", particularly those indicating psoriasis. Yet, although non-contagious, the latter bore the stigma of *ṣāra'at*, since they could not always be clearly distinguished from certain serious and contagious conditions. They were not subject to strict isolation, but were banned from the Sanctuary or Temple and thus remained under priestly supervision.

Moreover, chronic psoriasis can give rise to serious acute complications; these are not only potentially infectious, but may still more easily be mistaken for contagious bejel or leprosy. Such a case of psoriasis was then proclaimed as "unclean" and was subject to strict isolation but, if the complication remitted, it was once again considered as "clean".

Such a differentiation of *ṣāra'at* into "unclean" and "clean" would not only guard against the risk of mistaken diagnosis ("false negative" assessment); it would also obviate the danger of "false positive" categorization. Aiming to be as "fail-safe" as possible, it takes into account doubtful cases of both kinds.[84]

Thus the stated aim of all the "purity laws"—to distinguish the "unclean" from the "clean"—is treated in Leviticus 13 as differentiating conditions thought to be physically "contagious", or potentially so, from those not considered as such.[85] In view of the danger of contagion to the public, this served as a system of control that was not only rational and effective but also extraordinarily humane. Although rigid in form, the leniency of its provisions is striking, particularly when compared with the measures outlined in Numbers 5:2–3.

Nor is there any Biblical evidence that isolation was intended as punishment; it was related solely to physical contagion. Similarly, according to Leviticus 14, the atonement rites mandatory before the sufferer could be fully discharged were not linked to isolation, but to the possible moral "contagion". Thus the "medical", legal and ritual connotations merge in a concept of *ṣāra'at* based on "contagion", in both the physical and spiritual sense.

The table on the following page summarizes the laws of *ṣāra'at* in the simple, standardized binary ("yes–no") form in which they are presented in Leviticus 13. But it must once more be stressed that here the outcome has been interpreted in terms of modern medical "diagnoses", which were cer-

---

[84]However, according to Grmek, *Diseases in the Ancient Greek World*, 161, in Leviticus 13 signs of "one or even a few diseases that have serious consequences for the affected person and those around him" (which include leprosy, but not bejel) "*have been confused*" with those of certain skin diseases that are "relatively benign", such as psoriasis and vitiligo (my italics). He therefore concludes that "if such a practical definition... also includes some harmless skin diseases, isn't this because it seemed preferable to err in overestimating its severity, rather than risk the consequences of dangerous diseases?"

[85]Hulse, "The Nature of Biblical 'Leprosy'," 92, similarly considers that Leviticus 13 aims to distinguish *ṣāra'at* from other diseases that it may "superficially" resemble. However, like many others today, he defines *ṣāra'at* as representing conditions exhibiting scaly skin lesions, essentially psoriasis, but also certain banal skin diseases. He specifically excludes leprosy and does not mention bejel.

Verses in Leviticus 13	white hair	deeper than skin	unclean	*Modern Interpretation*	
				Disease	*Contagious*
9–11 18–20 24–25	+	+	+	bejel	+
43–46	(+)/ –	+	+	(bejel)/ leprosy	+
6	+	–	–	? vitiligo	–
12–13 17	–	–	–	chronic psoriasis	–
14–16	–	+	+	acute, general-ized pustular psoriasis	+/–
4–6 7–8 22–23 26–28	–	+	+	? cutaneous leishman-iasis, including diffuse type	(infectious) +

Table 1: Binary Presentation of Main Skin Signs of *Ṣāra'at* According to Leviticus 13, with a Modern Interpretation

tainly not comprehended at the time. The priests did not consider the syndromes in the form of specific "diseases", but in the language of ritual and law.

Thus the Biblical term *ṣāra'at* does not itself represent a "diagnosis" of any specific medical condition. Moreover, since the assessments were effected only on the basis of lesions that were both early and visible, the criteria intentionally omitted many of the characteristic clinical features that generally only become manifest when the disease is well advanced. Such signs, which help to confirm the "diagnosis", include the facial destruction of bejel and the cutaneous anaesthesia and *leonine facies* of leprosy. These sophisticated aspects of the concept of *ṣāra'at* have so far been little appreciated. On the contrary, they have reinforced the modern tendency to belittle its "medical" basis.

Some readers may feel that even this dualistic interpretation of Biblical *ṣāraʿat* smacks too much of "medical materialism". It would seem, however, desirable to consider both interpretations as equally valid, according to the circumstances of the case. Although, according to the Bible, *ṣāraʿat* was in general inflicted for sin, its practical rulings on the matter are based on the fear of contagion.

Epilogue

With the fall of the Second Temple in AD 70, the priestly caste of Israel ceased to function and thus no longer handled *ṣāraʿat*. This must have resulted in the loss of that accumulation of empirical knowledge and experience in this field, which the priests had transmitted orally from one generation to the other.[86] As seen from the Mishnah (Tractate *Negaʿim*) and allied writings, the Sages and Rabbis did their best, at great length, to explain the brief guidelines represented by Leviticus 13.[87] Even so, it seems impossible today to interpret their attempts on any rational medical basis.[88] This is not surprising, since, as has been seen, the specific medical problems of the Exodus had long been superseded. Thus the entire system now was superfluous and eventually was totally discarded.

A concept of physical contagion, however, does seem to underlie all the so-called "purity laws" of Leviticus 11–15, in view of the cryptic Biblical pronouncement that these aim "to distinguish the unclean from the clean". Here, an attempt has been made to develop this interpretation with regard to Leviticus 13 and 14, which deal essentially with certain skin lesions categorized in the Bible as *ṣāraʿat*.

No consensus yet exists regarding the meaning of this Hebrew term, although its usual translation as "leprosy" has been long and widely disputed. It is postulated here that this additional concept refers to the early skin manifestations of certain contagious, chronic, endemic diseases that affected the Israelites during and after the Exodus from Egypt. These signs are particularly applicable to bejel (endemic treponematosis), a highly contagious and

[86] However, according to Hulse (ibid., 94) the laws of Leviticus 13 would never have fallen into disuse had they been effective against contagion. (He therefore concludes that they were directed solely against "cultic uncleanness").

[87] J. Neusner, *A History of the Mishnaic Law of Purities*, Part 8, *Negaʿim* (Leiden: Brill, 1975), 244–5 and *passim*.

[88] Michman, "Leprosy," col. 38.

mutilating disease that might have threatened the very existence of the Israelites during their sojourn in the desert. Centuries later, after they were settled in Canaan, the rules were possibly adapted to leprosy (Hansen's disease). Such chronic contagious conditions were pronounced as both *ṣāra'at* and "unclean", and were subjected to isolation until recovery or death supervened.

Yet, throughout the Old Testament, the term *ṣāra'at* seems also to be applied to the skin signs of certain non-contagious and relatively harmless diseases, particularly chronic psoriasis. This category comprised certain chronic skin lesions that could easily be confused with the contagious conditions that were classed as "unclean". Hence they were considered as "potentially" contagious, and although they were pronounced as *ṣāra'at*, they were considered as "clean" and not isolated. They were excluded only from the Sanctuary or Temple, thereby remaining under priestly supervision.

Leviticus 13 may thus be interpreted as a system for the control of certain contagious endemic diseases that presented with characteristic skin lesions. The system of early identification was simple enough to be administered by the priests, who alone could enforce the regulations. Yet it not only prevented "false negative" assessments, but also—from an extraordinarily humane point of view—minimized the risk of "false positive" identification and isolation. The actual differentiation of *ṣāra'at* into "unclean" and "clean" and the grounds for isolation were thus based on the criterion of physical contagion; contrary to many traditional interpretations, they bore no moral connotation. However, since both forms of *ṣāra'at* were generally inflicted for lack of faith in God, this concept must also have involved moral or spiritual "contagion", as reflected in Leviticus 14.

7

Did the Greeks Have a Word for It? Contagion and Contagion Theory in Classical Antiquity

Vivian Nutton

Introduction

Few topics are so well-known and, at the same time, so baffling, as the observations and theories of the Greeks and Romans relating to contagion, and a speaker who has chosen to discourse on this theme risks boring an audience with the repetition of familiar examples as well as disappointing them with a conclusion that ends in uncertainty. Indeed, it might be argued that the world would be best served by a reprint or translation of the 1824 Göttingen dissertation of K. F. H. Marx, *Origines contagii*, an excellent collection of primary sources, which sets out with clarity and elegance the problems and possible solutions involved in a hunt for early ideas on contagion.[1] But since this most valuable of guides is only for the Latinate and, besides, is not easy to locate even in a large medical library, merely to reiterate its conclusions has a certain utility. In so doing, one must thread one's way through a complex of arguments that are frequently muddled together, and where the vagaries of translation have only added to the subsequent confusion. Indeed, at times authors seem unclear themselves just what they are trying to prove, mixing up discussions of terminology with those of aetiology, modern medical definitions with

[1] K. F. H. Marx, *Origines contagii* (Karlsruhe: D. R. Marx, 1824). One should note also the same author's *Additamenta ad origines contagii* (Karlsruhe: D. R. Marx, 1826), which is mainly concerned with the most recent manifestations of plague and with the latest discussions of its origin and treatment, but adds some extra references to ancient sources. Marx (1796–1877) went on to a chair of medicine at Göttingen, and to a distinguished career as a medical professor and medical historian.

ancient observations. In consequence, they have often come to totally different conclusions in their interpretation of a particular passage, and built some mighty theories on what may well turn out to be the flimsiest of foundations.

It will be best to begin with a few general statements on which all can agree. The first is that the words *contagio*, *contagium*, and related verbs and adjectives appear frequently in Latin, from at least the second century BC onwards, in contexts for which the English translation "contagion" would be appropriate. The words are used both metaphorically, of moral failings, and with a specific application to certain diseases, notably pest, phthisis, scabies, leprosy, and bleary eye, *lippitudo*. They encompass, although not necessarily all at the same time, notions of direct touch, of person-to-person transmission, and of the dangers of proximity, as well as of pollution and defilement.

Secondly, there is no single Greek word that is used so often and with such a specific application to disease as *contagio*.[2] In general the Greeks preferred to use such words as "share", "pass", and "receive", which emphasize the common illness rather than a particular method of transmission.[3]

The touch of *epaphe*

This is not to say that no such word existed, for Karl Sudhoff drew attention to an example in a papyrus, from the first century BC, of a slave girl who was sold not subject to any prior title, deed, or contract, and without any long-standing lesion, *epaphe*, weals, or hidden condition.[4] Etymologically, *epaphe* derives from the Greek verb "to touch", and thus offers a close parallel to the Latin *contagio*. Its occurrence here, sandwiched between other words of medical significance, suggests that it has medical rather than legal connotations, and the appearance in similar slave contracts of the phrase "free from the sacred disease and *epaphe*" may likewise refer to an ailment rather than a legal

[2] I use *contagio* as this appears to be the earlier form of the word; *contagium* is found more often in verse. The two are interchangeable in meaning and context.

[3] Greek ideas on "sharing" the disease have been recently studied by Karl-Heinz Leven, "Miasma und Metadosis. Antike Vorstellungen von Ansteckung," *Medizin, Gesellschaft und Geschichte, Jahrbuch des Instituts für Geschichte der Medizin der Robert Bosch Stiftung* 11 (1992): 43–73; *idem*, "Antike und Mittelalter," in F. Hoffmann, ed., *Infektologie. Diagnostik—Therapie—Prophylaxe. Handbuch und Atlas für Klinik und Praxis* (Augsburg: Ecomed, 1992), 1–16.

[4] Karl Sudhoff, "᾽Επαφή der Aussatz?," *Sudhoffs Archiv für Geschichte der Medizin* 21 (1929): 204–6, on P. Strasbourg 79.

charge.[5] Whether Sudhoff was right to identify this "touch" with leprosy, as opposed to other diseases where one might be "touched", or even contagious disease in general, is uncertain. What is most striking is that this word appears in a context of disease (whether physical or moral) only once outside this handful of legal texts, which, since Greek texts from the period before AD 600 outnumber Latin writings considerably, is a point of some significance, to which I shall return later.[6] But, lest we are carried away with the exciting prospect of *epaphe* as a Greek technical term for contagion, we should remember that it and its verb *ephaptein* simply mean "touch"; the prefix *epi-* intensifies the touching, and does not stress the sharing of the touch implicit in the Latin prefix *con-*. Nor is it immediately obvious who or what, in these legal texts, is doing the touching: it could be a diseased individual or a disease itself, for the Hippocratic Corpus refers to diseases that "touch" patients, and a glance at any Greek dictionary will show how non-medical authors like Sophocles and Thucydides used the same mode of expression for the behaviour of diseases.[7] To put it another way, Greek diseases regularly touched the sick; they were not, lexically speaking, usually *con*tagious.

There is, however, one author who employs *epaphe* in an unequivocally medical context; Plutarch, who in his *Table Talk*, written around AD 100, records the conversations of himself and his friends over dinner in Greece. They discuss the meaning of Homeric phrases, the propriety of philosophizing at table, and a variety of medical and natural-historical topics, ranging from whether women are naturally hotter or colder than men to the causes of thirst and the possible existence of new diseases. Doctors share in this learned chit-chat, and Plutarch is happy to report their theories, whether Methodist or Hippocratic. He himself is an interested amateur, with a competent understanding of the theoretical points at issue.

In Book V.7, his guests turn to the subject of "fascination", the evil eye. Most of them are sceptical of its very existence, but Mestrius Florus, an elderly ex-consul, quotes an earlier historian, Phylarchus, to the effect that

---

[5] H. G. Liddell, R. Scott, and H. S. Jones, *A Greek–English Lexicon*, rev. ed. (Oxford: Clarendon Press, 1968), 612, cite other papyri but suggest that the word means "legal claim".

[6] The word is used again in the context of contagion and infection by the Byzantine author George Scholarios (writing between 1459 and 1470), who compares the transmission of plague from city to city with that of a curse that touches and defiles. See M. H. Congourdeau, "La société byzantine face aux grandes pandémies," in *Maladie et société à Byzance*, ed. E. Patlagean (Spoleto: Centro italiano di studi sull'alto medioevo, 1993), 21–41, esp. 39.

[7] Sophocles, *Trachiniae*, 1010; Thucydides, *Hist.* II.48; J. H. Kühn and U. Fleischer, *Index hippocraticus* (Göttingen: Vandenhoeck und Ruprecht, 1986), I, 84.

the Palaeothebans, backwoodsmen from Pontus (modern N. Turkey), had the power to kill both adults and children with a single stare; those who were the recipients of such a stare, or were breathed upon, or merely addressed, wasted away and fell ill. Slave-traders in that region, Florus continues, confirm this story, which in itself is hardly surprising, for touching (*epaphe*) and *synanachrosis* provide an obvious starting point (*arche*) for disease—just as the introduction of eagle feathers into a mass of other feathers results in their putrefaction and dissolution. It is exactly the same with the human touch (*haphe*): sometimes it helps, sometimes it is fatal. One must accept that injury from the evil eye occurs, even if one cannot immediately track down its cause. Plutarch, ever the kind host, politely informs his guests that Florus has put them on the right path in pointing to "effluxes" (*aporrhoiai*) from the body as the cause. Smell, voice, and the flow of breath are portions of animals that are carried outwards and stimulate the senses of others whenever they are encountered. However unlikely at first sight, then, there is a scientific and, indeed, mechanistic explanation for the evil eye.

Synanachrosis

With this mechanistic explanation, I shall not yet be concerned, nor need much be said about the evil eye except that the discussion of contagion, sympathy, and the principle of action at a distance is frequently linked to the problem of explaining the evil eye. My immediate concern is with the words *epaphe* and *synanachrosis*. Both the succeeding example and the comment that the human touch may produce the same deleterious effect as an eagle's feather make it clear that Plutarch and Florus were referring to a physical contact, touching and *synanachrosis*, a noun found only here.

What does this rare word *synanachrosis* mean? Etymologically it is composed of a noun and two prefixes, *syn-*, "with", and *ana-*, which usually either indicates repetition or intensifies the action of the verb. The latter part of the word is related to *chros*, the Greek word for "flesh" or "colour", and to a root verb that means to dye, to touch, and, in the tragedians and in the Hippocratic *On Breaths*, to "pollute". Explaining "common" diseases, the author of *On Breaths* notes in Chapter 6 that "when the air is polluted/dyed/infected with miasmata that are hostile to human nature, humans fall ill; when the air is unsuitable for other types of living being, then they in turn fall ill". We have in *synanachrosis*, then, a word that etymologically corresponds to the

Latin *contagio*, containing both an element of touching and of sharing, and with a main root frequently associated with moral as well as physical illness.

The noun and its associated verbs are used by Plutarch in several passages, all of which, explicitly or implicitly, involve some form of association as well as transmission. Land animals by their kinship and cohabitation and by being "in contact" with human habits also learn to share in their food, their training, and their mimicry (*On Training Animals*, 975 E). One should be careful with one's children lest by associating (or "being in contact") with foreigners and those of bad habits they pick up some of their wickedness (*On Bringing Up Children*, 4 A). King Agis of Sparta was right to fear that foreigners "coming into contact" with his austere citizens would reproduce in them some of their alien luxury, effeminacy, and extravagance (*Agis* X.3).

Although Plutarch provides most examples of the noun and verb, he is not the earliest author to use the verb. That honour should perhaps go to an astronomer, Geminus of Rhodes, who is generally assumed to have lived around 70 BC.[8] In his *Introduction to Astronomy*, II.14, he briefly discusses the sympathy between the constellations, explaining it thus: "The emanation (*apophora*) and efflux (*aporrhoia*) that are produced from the particular property of each star must mingle and come into contact with the neighbouring signs."

The word is also used twice by a Roman writer, Florentinus, active around AD 230, who is quoted at length in the Greek *Geoponics*, a collection of passages on gardens and farming. Florentinus advises gardeners to cut down trees growing in a circle, for their roots "are damaged by becoming intertwined and in contact with the odours of figs and, even more, of wild figs and pomegranates." By contrast, a well-designed park will be a delight and a profitable concern, for "the ambient air, being in contact with the effluxes (*aporrhoiai*) from the plants, will make the property truly wholesome".[9]

Students of medical lexicography may wish to believe that the evidence I have so far put forward is enough to prove that, as far as contagion is con-

[8] The verb is used by the historian Diodorus Siculus at the end of the first century BC, *Hist.* III.16, in his description of the way in which Egyptians prepare a fishpaste, trampling sun-dried fish and thornberries together on a smooth stone until, by "mingling them together", everything becomes glutinous. Diodorus' source for this is the earlier (about 120 BC) historian Agatharchides, and the verb may well have been used by the latter.

[9] *Geoponics* VI.ii.9, X.i.1. Save for the example in Diodorus quoted earlier, the latter is the only surviving passage in which the verb carries with it positive connotations. The *Thesaurus linguae graecae*, s.v. *synanachronnumi*, cites later Byzantine evidence for the meaning "to dye".

cerned, the Greeks did indeed have a word for it—and perhaps two, *epaphe* and *synanachrosis*. But the very rarity of both of these words in surviving authors is striking in comparison with the common appearance of their Latin equivalents in a variety of texts and contexts from the second century BC onwards. It shows that, at the very least, Greek and Latin authors each preferred a different vocabulary of metaphor.

Neat proof of this can be found in those instances where the Latin has *contagium* or *contagio* and a Greek translation or equivalent version survives. According to Du Cange and the *Thesaurus linguae latinae*, the Latin words are never glossed by a direct equivalent that incorporates in a single word both halves of the Latin. Sometimes a totally different word or concept is used, notably *miasma*, or "diseases of proximity"; sometimes, as in a translation into Greek from Virgil, *Eclogues* I,50, *mala vicini pecoris contagia* ("the evil contagion of a nearby beast"), the compound word is simplified into "the touch of a sick sheep". The Septuagint translators of Leviticus 13 and 14 had no difficulty in rendering directly into Greek "the touch of leprosy" (Jerome's later *tactus leprae*); by contrast, at Numbers 19:18, where Jerome has *homines huiuscemodi contagione pollutos* ("men polluted with a touch of this sort"), the Greek has a totally different version "on those persons whosoever might be there, and on him who has touched the human bone". The latter is either a bad translation or the result of following a different or defective text. In brief, nowhere is there found a direct Greek translation corresponding to *contagio*, *contactus*, even though it would have been easy to form a calque by using a word for touch along with the prefix *syn-* ("with"), either on its own or in combination with other prefixes, especially when, as we have seen, at least one such word already existed and might have been used. To put it another way, and one that has wider implications, Latin writers very often use *contagio/-um* in contexts, and even occasionally in identical passages, where the Greek is not so specific. Greeks share or pollute, Latins touch.

The perils of proximity

Having identified two possible Greek words for contagion, neither, as far as we can tell, widely used, we perhaps should end this enquiry. But if we forsake the purely lexicographical definition implicit in the title of this paper, then we are only at the very beginning of a proper investigation.

Once again, we can start from agreed data. Already by the end of the fifth century BC Greek writers, mainly in Athens, were aware that in certain diseases those in proximity to the sick were themselves liable to fall ill in the same way. In his famous description of the Great Plague of Athens in 430 BC, the historian Thucydides, himself a sufferer, expressly mentioned that those who attended the sick were most in danger of falling ill and dying: "the doctors were themselves most likely to die inasmuch as they were the most faithful attendants of the sick". A few lines later on he remarked that men died like sheep, having become "filled with disease through attending on one another. . . .if they came to visit, they were likely to die, especially those who still retained a trace of goodness. Honour made them unsparing of themselves in their attendance in their friends' houses, where even the members of the family were at last worn out by the moans of the dying and succumbed to the immense evil." A similar implication may also be found in his concluding statement that the plague was distributed most widely in Athens, and after that in the regions that were most densely populated.[10]

Here is ample proof that the phenomenon of contagion, in the broad sense of a disease of proximity, was noticed and specifically commented on by a literate and thinking observer. But one should also be careful. Thucydides does not include any indication of the method of contagion, except, apparently, that it involved some form of contact, direct or indirect, with the sick. He does not even go so far as to imply that this was the major way in which the disease was transmitted.[11]

A similar perception of the likelihood that those who tended the sick would themselves fall ill of the same disease comes in the *Aegineticus*, a speech delivered a few years later by the orator Isocrates before a jury on the island of Aegina. Appearing for the defence, Isocrates tells in grim detail of the last days of Thrasylochus, a sufferer from *phthoe* (probably tuberculosis) bereft of carers, save for a single slave and the defendant. The few friends who dared come near declared that they feared for the defendant's life as well as that of the patient. They urged him to leave at once, for, they said, "most of those who treat this disease are themselves killed by it too." The courage of Isocrates' client, and the propriety of the legacy bequeathed to him, are enhanced by the

[10] Respectively, *Hist.* II.47, 51, 54.

[11] A. J. Holladay and J. F. C. Poole, "Thucydides and the Plague of Athens," *Classical Quarterly*, N. S. 29 (1979): 282–300, esp. 296–300, are somewhat excessive in their claims for what an understanding of contagion on the part of doctors might have done, had they read their Thucydides carefully. It is clear from Thucydides' account that the perception of the danger of propinquity was not his alone. See now Simon Hornblower, *A Commentary on Thucydides*, I (Oxford: Clarendon Press, 1991), 316–18.

apparently universal recognition of the danger he was facing. How more deserving the anonymous defendant than the sister who sent each day to find out how Thrasylochus was, but who did not think it wise to pay even the briefest of visits from her refuge in the nearest mainland port! In this speech we have a clear recognition of the likelihood of person-to-person transmission of one illness, and Marx's list of authors, both Greek and Latin, historians, moralists, and theologians, confirms beyond any doubt that the notion that proximity to the sick might be dangerous, particularly in cases of "plague" and phthisis, was widespread throughout Antiquity, among both Greeks and Latins.[12]

What is less clear is any ancient understanding of why proximity should be dangerous. That question is not raised in our extant sources before the pseudo-Aristotelian *Problems*, a composite work, difficult to date or to ascribe to any single author, but unlikely to predate 320 BC. In Book I.7 (859b15–20), the writer wonders why the plague (*loimos*) alone "fills" those who come close to those who are under treatment for it, and suggests that this is because the plague is a disease common to all, i.e. not specific to any single humoral mixture. Anyone can thus be quickly "caught" by the inflammatory matter produced by the disease and transmitted by the patient. In Book VII.4 (886b3–8), the question is asked why those in proximity to sufferers from certain diseases "are caught," whereas no one ever becomes healthy through proximity to health.[13]

The problem of proximity is further considered at Book VII.8 (887a22–887b1), where the diseases that are caught from attending to the sick are specified as phthisis, ophthalmia, and *psora* (scabies), but not dropsy, fevers, or apoplexy. The author then wonders if this is the result of a specific quality in the eye that assimilates itself to what it sees, or because phthisis corrupts the breath, as in plague. As for *psora*, it, like leprosy, affects the surface of the body, and causes the production, and transmission, of a glutinous discharge. Dry or deep-seated diseases cannot be caught in this way, for they are neither sticky nor confined to the skin.

[12] One might also note the stories of corpses being hurled into besieged towns. Cf. M. D. Grmek, "Les ruses de guerre biologiques dans l'Antiquité," *Revue des études grecques* 92 (1979): 140–63.

[13] The latter sentiment is also expressed at XXIX.10 (951a3–5), which contrasts the lack of improvement in health with the increase in virtue by association with the virtuous. To the first question the response is that health is a state, not an active movement like disease; to the second, that physical health cannot be imitated by the soul.

The same question and the same explanation recur, almost unchanged, in the collection of *Problems* ascribed to Alexander of Aphrodisias and compiled no earlier than AD 200 and perhaps two centuries later. The problem of the transmissibility of disease contrasted with that of health is referred specifically to ophthalmia (I.35, probably the result of combining two separate questions from the Aristotelian collection). The longer question about phthisis, *psora*, and ophthalmia is, however, repeated almost word for word at II.42. However, the question on plague in this collection (I.88) is rather different, for it asks why "in a plague situation" some die and others live. The response concentrates on the receptivity of an individual humoral constitution to putrid air and compares the spread of plague to that of a fire in a field; straw burns fast, but some trees remain almost unscathed.

The sort of explanation offered in these *Problems*, both sets of which are firmly Peripatetic in orientation, differs from that already noted in the discussion of *synanachrosis*. There is no reference to effluxes and emanations, and the Aristotelian problem concerned with the evil eye, Book XX.34 (926a20–31), deals only with its possible cure by eating rue. A Peripatetic, or genuinely Aristotelian, source for the theory of *synanachrosis* is thus somewhat unlikely. An origin in Greek philosophy, however, is certain, for the word is formed like a technical term, as are both emanation and effluxion.

Plutarch provides a possible clue, for in his description of the debate on new disease (*Symp.* VIII.9) he ascribes to the "Democriteans" a theory of effluxes of bodies from the worlds outside our own, which often result in the onset of plagues and unusual diseases. On another occasion (*Symp.* VI.8), he makes a doctor, Cleomenes, talk of an emanation from dried figs and apples that produces heartburn and dizziness. That such ideas were associated with an atomist or quasi-atomist view of the human body is likely from the fact that a similar belief in the importance of emanations in the causation of disease was ascribed to Asclepiades of Bithynia (around 95 BC) by the (much later) Cassius the Iatrosophist,[14] and is further associated with Asclepiades and the somewhat later Alexander Philalethes (fl. AD 15) by the author of the last section of the Anonymus Londinensis papyrus.[15] Both of these physicians

[14] Cassius Iatrosophistes, *Problems* 40, with the discussion in J. T. Vallance, *The Lost Theory of Asclepiades of Bithynia* (Oxford: Clarendon Press, 1990), 86–8.

[15] The author of Anon. Lon. XXI–end is not himself so firm a believer in *apophorai*, but his own doctrinal adherence is not entirely clear. The word *apophora* is not found in Galen;

favoured a mechanistic view of the body that was akin to those of Epicurus and Democritus.[16] A link between the theory of contagion and atomism, whether Democritean, Epicurean, or Asclepiadean, is at least plausible, and would help to explain some of the discrepancies between the Greek and Latin uses of contagion.[17] Latin authors of the first century BC, most notably Cicero and Lucretius, are far more informative about Epicureanism than what survives in Greek from the same period, and Epicureanism seems to have enjoyed a certain reputation in late-Republican Rome. In medicine, the quasi-atomist theories of Asclepiades were transformed by his successors into Methodism, a medical doctrine that had great success in Rome and with which Plutarch was acquainted through his friend, the doctor Philo.[18] Plutarch's own philosophical eclecticism and wide learning also explain why he should put forward views on disease and the evil eye that involve emanations and effluxes and are not mentioned by the later dominant Aristotelian or Platonist philosophers—or by Galen, so resolutely hostile to Methodists and Epicureans.

Contagion and Later Methodism

Indeed, it may be no coincidence that the only surviving strictly medical sources to refer to contagion are the fifth-century Latin Methodist writer, Caelius Aurelianus, and his contemporary, the Methodist-influenced Theodore Priscian. The latter merely declares (*Log.* 59) that a cough can cause trouble through proximity, "as if by a sort of contagion". Caelius Aurelianus, the compiler of a large work on *Acute and Chronic Diseases* heavily dependent

---

and *aporrhoia* only twice, both times applied to the effluxes from the human body, not in any cosmological or physiological context. This may indicate that the theory of *apophorai* (and their consequence) was not accepted by Hippocratics in general, but cf. below, 156.

[16]For Alexander, cf. H. von Staden, *Herophilus: the Art of Medicine in Early Alexandria* (Cambridge: Cambridge University Press, 1989), 532–5.

[17]A. Thivel, "La dénomination des maladies chez Lucrèce," in G. Sabbah, ed., *Le latin médical: la constitution d'un langage scientifique, Actes du IIIe colloque international "Textes médicaux latins antiques," St. Etienne, 1989, Mémoires du Centre Jean Palerne* 10 (1991): 242–56, argues for Epicurus as the link between Democritus and the theory of "seeds of disease" in Lucretius, and as a possible source for this type of explanation in terms of contagion. For Methodist involvement, cf. my "The Seeds of Disease," *Medical History* 27 (1983): 1–34, at 8–11; repr. with identical pagination as Chapter XI in my *From Democedes to Harvey: Studies in the History of Medicine* (London: Variorum, 1988).

[18]S. T. Teodorsson, *A Commentary on Plutarch's Table Talks*, II (Gothenburg: Almqvist and Wiksell, 1990), provides a general survey of Plutarch's scientific interests and an exposition of the main points at issue.

on the writings of the Greek Soranus of Ephesus (fl. AD 100), is somewhat more informative, but, as we shall see, none of the six instances in which he uses *contagio/-um* is without its problems.[19]

At *Chron.* I.129, Caelius derides a variety of exotic remedies used for epilepsy, arguing that they cannot be justified by the notion of "occult causes" nor can they have come into medicine *ex aliqua contagione siue tentatione, ut Empirici volunt.* To translate the word here as "contagion" makes no sense, and no one has ever attempted to do so. Ingeborg Pape, the most recent translator, understands the phrase to mean "through chance or experience, as the Empiricists want", but there is no other example of *contagio* meaning "chance" and emendation to *ex aliquo contingenti* is unsatisfactory.[20] Drabkin offers a very different rendering, "on the basis of trial and experience". This is much closer to Empiricist doctrine, and has the advantage that *sive tentatione* is treated as a gloss on *contagione*, a common stylistic feature of Caelius' writing that reflects a method of translating an underlying Greek substrate.[21] But against this, it can be objected that *contagio* cannot mean "trial" either. Emendation is essential. We must either read *cogitatione*, "reasoning", and apply the qualification "as the Empirics want" only to "or experience": if so, Caelius is claiming that these remedies have been approved neither by reason nor by experience. The alternative, and better, course is to follow the emendation proposed in the margin of the 1567 edition of Caelius and read *cognitione*, the technical term for a legal trial. The text then corresponds to an original Greek *peira*, to Drabkin's version, and to a typical mannerism of Caelius and other late-Latin translators, the rendering of a single technical Greek word by two near-synonyms. Whichever emendation is preferred, the word *contagio* must disappear.[22]

---

[19] For Theodore, see P. Migliorini, "Elementi Metodici in Teodoro Prisciano," in *Les écoles médicales à Rome*, ed. P. Mudry and J. Pigeaud (Geneva: Droz, 1991), 231–40; for Caelius, J. Pigeaud, "Pro Caelio Aureliano," *Mémoires du Centre Jean Palerne* 3 (1982): 105–18.

[20] Pape's translation accompanies the edition of Gerhard Bendz in *Corpus medicorum latinorum*, VI (Berlin: Akademie Verlag, 1990–3), that of I. E. Drabkin his edition (Chicago: University of Chicago Press, 1950). Both translations are cited by the chapter and section number only.

[21] Cf. M. E. Vazquez Bujan, "Compréhension, traduction, adaptation: De Caelius Aurélianus aux traductions du VIe siècle," in G. Sabbah, ed., *Le latin médical*, 87–97.

[22] The passage is omitted from the collection of fragments in K. Deichgräber, *Die griechische Empirikerschule* (Berlin and Zurich: Weidmann'sche Buchhandlung, 1965), but cf. frags. 146–8.

A few sections later, at I.149, Caelius reports the views of "some people" who believe that in trying to distinguish cases of epilepsy and mania one should also take account of the "quality of the diseases as they come to the body, for these often attack the body by a kind of *contagio*". Even so, says Caelius, this will not produce a totally secure differential diagnosis, for although sleeplessness, anxiety and the like may well occur in those about to fall prey to epilepsy and mental disorder, they may not all be present in any one attack, and there may be other signs that the authors have not mentioned. In this passage Caelius may be referring to some form of transmitted disease, but this is far from clear, and any relationship to epilepsy and mental diseases is at best indirect. Drabkin translates *contagio* simply as "external contact", with no connotation of contagion.

More straightforward is Caelius' quotation (*Chron.* I.57) from a Hippocratic "Silimachus" who reported that in Rome many people were affected by the nightmare feelings of the incubus through "a sort of plague-like contagion". Three points are of interest here. The first is that there is an implicit link made between contagion and *lues*, although in the discussion of *lues* itself at *Ac.* I.12 the word *contagio* does not occur and the disease is defined only as one that arises from a common cause.[23] Secondly, as in the previous quotation, Caelius is associating what some considered a part-physical, part-mental condition with contagion, although for both conditions he posits a purely physical cause. Thirdly, this opinion is ascribed to a Hippocratic physician, Lysimachus of Cos, a Greek writer of the second century BC, which might suggest that he had used a word for contagion.[24] But its appearance here could simply reflect a Latin way of rendering a Greek original, and is not evidence for a Hippocratic theory of contagion.

At *Ac.* III.52 Caelius reports that weaklings are harder to cure of a stroke than the strong, women than men, the old and the young than those in the prime of life, the unhealthy than the healthy, and those who have been previously touched by (the?) disease than those who have never been "wounded

[23]Contrast Pontius, *Vita Cypriani* 9, who describes the *lues dira* of 252 as a *contagium*, and bewails the folly of those who thought that by removing a near-dead sufferer from their presence they would also remove death itself.

[24]Both here and at *Ac.* III.138, Salimachus, the name is obviously wrong; it is a matter of judgement whether the error is due to Caelius (or his source), in which case "Sili-/Salimachus" should be left in the text, or, perhaps more likely, to the process of transmission, in which case the text in both places should be emended to "Lysimachus," as Wellmann saw. Pape/Bendz print and translate Sili-, Sali- without comment; Drabkin notes the problem only in his index, 1002, 1008.

by the *contagio* of the disease". If, as seems likely, Caelius's comments refer specifically to stroke, and not to diseases in general, one can only applaud the clinical judgement that regards a patient suffering a second stroke as extremely hard to cure. The Latin word can then hardly be translated as "contagion", in the modern sense of the term, but, following up the metaphor implied in "wounded", it signifies merely the touch, or the assault, of the disease. There is no suggestion of proximity or transmissibility.[25]

The same phrase *contagione sauciari* reappears at *Chron.* IV.13, in a discussion of "elephantiasis" (i.e. leprosy, not the modern disease of the same name). Although, from the context, which talks of the segregation of sufferers, it is extremely tempting to translate the phrase as "wounded by the contagion of this disease", its occurrence at *Ac.* III.52 and possibly *Chron.* I.149, and perhaps the author's familiarity with the biblical "touch of leprosy", might indicate that Caelius is referring simply to the touch of the disease rather than its transmissibility. But there is no doubt that Caelius knows of authors who strongly believe that leprosy is spread by contact, and who advocate tough preventative measures. In their view, if leprosy appears in a town previously free of it, the leper should be imprisoned (*cludendum)*, if he is a stranger;[26] if a citizen, he should be exiled to an inland and cooler climate until health is restored, in order to prevent others from "being wounded by the *contagio* of the disease". But that, says Caelius, is alien to the humane spirit of medicine.

Neither in Caelius nor elsewhere in the Latin tradition, although it refers far more often than the Greek to the "contagion" of some diseases, is there any discussion of the actual process of transmission. Nevertheless, as well as explanations for "plague" in terms of changes in the atmosphere and the poisoning of the air, several authors stress the importance of direct contact. Even if the etymological explanation of Isidore of Seville—"Contagion, from *contingo*, "I touch", because whoever one touches is polluted"—is discounted

[25] Cf. Drabkin, 833 n. 4, querying the specificity of the reference. The word may have this meaning of "touch" or "assault" at I.149, and it would seem to be used in this general sense at *Ac.* II.198, where it is ascribed to one of the founders of Methodism, Thessalus (fl. AD 60). But since Thessalus himself probably wrote in Greek, the appearance of the word here may be due to the translator.

[26] Drabkin, 822, suspected the text here, and suggested *excludendum* ("removed") or the even harsher *caedendum* ("be killed"). But the latter is an otherwise unprecedented punishment for leprosy, and, if an emendation is required, *secludendum* is palaeographically more likely, and removal beyond the boundary of the city an apt reaction. But given the vagueness of Caelius' report, emendation is perhaps unwarranted, for there is no evidence that these procedures were ever carried out. Benz, 782, accepts *caedendum* without comment.

as the mere speculation of a lexicographer, it was by no means a foolish guess. The historian Livy, about AD 10, had described how those who treated the sick themselves spread the disease by touch (*contactus*, XXV.xxvi.8). Earlier in his *History*, at III.vi.3, he had expressed the same sentiments in a different way by using the word *contagio*.[27] An oration ascribed to the historian Sallust and written no later than the early first century AD uses rabies as an example of a disease spread by touch (*contactu*). Pliny the Elder in his discussion of the new diseases of the early Roman Empire also describes how the *contagio* of a skin disease called lichen or mentagra was introduced into Rome by a government official returning from the Eastern provinces: once in Rome it spread very fast through kissing (XXVI.iii.3). A later reviser of Pliny's medical sections put it more bluntly still; sufferers from lichen should not kiss, for the contact is extremely dangerous.[28] But, generally, the Latin writers simply use the words *contagio/-um*, both literally and metaphorically, without in any way revealing how, in their view, contagion works. The word itself carries an implication of a mechanical process of disease transmission by direct touch, but this implication may not always have been understood or intended, and should not be read back into every occurrence of the words.

Metaphor and the tyranny of modern medicine

Bedevilling many discussions of ancient theories of contagion lurks the belief that, in many ways, the ancients thought as we do today, and that modern conceptions of disease can be discovered, or at least are prefigured, in ancient sources. The worthy Marx did not collect his evidence as a piece of antiquarianism, but, as the first half of his book shows, as a contribution to contemporary debates on epidemics and their diffusion. His *Additamenta*, published two years later, is largely concerned with reviewing the relevance of his ancient sources to the very latest debates on contagion, as he and his fellow medical men understood it. Likewise, it is no coincidence that the discoveries of Pasteur, Koch, and other bacteriologists in the second half of the nineteenth century produced a renewal of interest in Fracastoro and in his classical predecessors, or that the focus of these new debates should have shifted from that

---

[27] The *Thesaurus linguae latinae*, col. 624, cites Livy IV.xxx.8: *volgatique contactu in homines morbi* ("the diseases were spread among men by contact"). Some editors reject *contactu* as a marginal gloss, but even if they are right, the gloss itself is very early, before AD 600, and can serve as an example of a classical belief in the spread of a disease by direct contact.

[28] *Physica Plinii* I.18, ed. Önnerfors.

of Marx. Contagion, having been redefined by the bacteriologists, was now sought anew—and not found before the sixteenth century. Conversely, translators, familiar with the language of modern medicine, eagerly employed it to elucidate their Greek and Latin sources. Contagion, pathogens, and germs infiltrated the thought world of the ancients, and Aristotle was made to speak as if addressing the Royal Society of Medicine.[29]

This process was facilitated by the very similarity of some of the words involved, not least the misleading pair of infection and contagion. As we have already seen, *contagio* cannot always be translated as "contagion", and even when it can, there is never the implication that what is being transmitted from person to person is a disease entity. What passes is an emanation, an effluxion, a breath, a poison, a putrid effusion, an excrement, or a miasma. There were also, as I have argued elsewhere, medical writers who talked of "seeds of disease" in a context of "new" diseases, but the precise meaning of this metaphor is hard to define, and was at best a minority view. Even among those who believed in this theory, their idea of specific diseases may have been considerably different from that of modern scholars influenced by the triumphs of bacteriology.[30]

Nor did the Latin word *inficere* carry the connotations that "infection" has for us. *Inficere*, as Danielle Gourévitch and Mirko Grmek have often insisted, is a metaphor that derives from the dyeing of cloth.[31] Similarly, the Greek words associated with the root "chros", mentioned at the beginning of this paper, have the same associations. Just as cloth, once dyed, takes on a different colour, and a small spot of dye gradually spreads over the adjacent fabric, so too the ambient air or the body, once "infected", becomes different from what it was before. It is an all-embracing process, whose end result is clear, even if

[29]At *Problems* VII.8, Forster's Oxford translation uses the word "contagion" three times, "contact" three times, and "infect" once. None is strictly present in the original Greek, and the result is a misleading modernization.

[30]Nutton, "The Seeds of Disease"; Owsei Temkin, "An Historical Analysis of the Concept of Infection," in his *The Double Face of Janus* (Baltimore: Johns Hopkins University Press, 1977), 456–71.

[31]M. D. Grmek, "Le concept d'infection dans l'Antiquité et au Moyen Age," *Travaux de l'Académie jougoslave* 384 (1980): 9–55; *idem*, "Les vicissitudes des notions d'infection, de contagion et de germe dans la médecine antique," *Mémoires du Centre Jean Palerne* 5 (1984): 53–70; Danielle Gourévitch, "Les faux-amis dans la compréhension et la traduction des textes médicaux de l'Antiquité," *Mémoires du Centre Jean Palerne* 3 (1982): 189–91; *idem*, "Peut-on employer le mot d'*infection* dans les traductions françaises de textes latins?," *Mémoires du Centre Jean Palerne* 5 (1984): 49–52.

the means by which the process is achieved are not. One can see the pustules of smallpox, and smell the putrid air of a sick room, even if one cannot agree on precisely how they came into existence. "Infecting" and "touching" are just two of the metaphors invoked to describe this process, and, as with any metaphor, their exact strength is hard to determine without a very clear context. What is beyond doubt, however, is that those who employed them did not understand contagion as it came to be defined in the late nineteenth century.

Both words also occupy the same semantic field as others that, to a modern scientist, are totally incompatible. Bilingual glossaries link *contagio* with Greek words for miasmata, pollution, defilement, amd sympathetic disease, or with other Latin words for defilement such as *coinquinatio.* In a widespread disease, the air, according to the writer of the Hippocratic *On Breaths,* "enmiasmed with diseased miasms" enters the body (V.9; VI.2) and becomes harmful to humans when it is "dyed with miasms hostile to human nature". The author of *On the Nature of Man* declares that the cause of epidemic disease is the air we breathe becoming possessed of a "diseased excrement" (9). The same vocabulary is used of medical, moral, and religious infection, and it is hard, if not impossible, to determine the precise register in which a given phrase is uttered.[32] Plato (*Phaedo* 67a2–6) talks of the effect of the soul's association with the body in terms that apply equally to disease and to religious pollution, and, as Glenn Most has recently argued, scholars have had great difficulty in deciding just how the Greek words, which etymologically relate to "filled with", are to be translated.[33] One can contaminate the atmosphere with sin as well as with noxious breath, and the polluted sinner, like the sufferer from phthisis, brings also a cloud of pollution that might affect, or infect, those who draw near.[34] Indeed, the emphasis in tragedy on the dire consequences of association with, and particularly of touching, an individual sinner might

[32]Fundamental is R. Parker, *Miasma: Pollution and Purification in Early Greek Religion* (Oxford: Clarendon Press, 1983).

[33]Glenn R. Most, "A Cock for Asclepius," *Classical Quarterly* N. S. 43 (1993): 96–111, at 101. Cf. Marx, *Origines contagii,* 143–6, for a list of words used in both medical and religious contexts. Mrs. E. M. Craik drew my attention to Sophocles, *Philoctetes,* 520: "when you are filled (fed up) with the disease by its [continual] presence".

[34]There were also those who believed that some diseases that some Hippocratic authors treated by physical means on the basis of physical explanation were in fact the result of some pollution and to be treated by means appropriate to religious pollution (*Sacred Disease* 2–4).

seem much closer to modern ideas of contagion than the ancient medical view that usually interposes an aerial *miasma* as intermediary.[35]

A similar collocation of medical, religious, and moral meanings accompanies *contagio.* In Ennius, *Plays*, 350, and Cato, *On Agriculture*, 132, two of the earliest examples of the word, it carries overtones of pollution beyond the mere act of touching. It is a favourite of the historian Livy, who applies it to lust for booty, or military glory, and who praises the Greek inhabitants of Marseilles (*Hist.* XXXVII.liv.22) for preserving their morals, laws, and intellectual life free of the contagion of the native Gauls who surrounded them—unlike the fierce Gauls who, having once conquered Galatia (central Turkey), were reduced to peaceful and unwarlike peasants by the fertility of the soil and the gentle behaviour of its inhabitants, a prime example of the contagious effects of indiscipline and local custom (*Hist.* XXXVIII.xvii.18). Livy describes the great—and still unexplained—Bacchanalia conspiracy of 186 BC in lurid terms. This pestilential evil, which he views as an enormous threat to the Roman state, spread from Etruria to Rome as if by the contagion of disease (*Hist.* XXXIX.ix.1). Later on, the evil of debt-inspired rebellion travelled throughout the Perrhaebian region of Greece by a contagion like that of phthisis (*Hist.* XLII.v.7). Physical and moral diseases are almost interchangeable. Whether pagan or Christian, heretic or libertine, the views of one's opponents are characterized by the metaphors of disease and contagion, of pollution and contamination. Pliny the Younger, writing to the emperor Trajan around AD 110, describes (*Epist.* X.xcvi.9) how the "contagion of Christian superstition" has penetrated even to the small towns of his province of Bithynia (NW Turkey).[36] Two hundred years later, around AD 334, the Christian emperor Constantine used the same language to denote paganism: in a letter to the cities of Umbria (central Italy) he allowed them to build a temple in his honour and to hold games, provided only that "the temple dedicated to our name shall not be polluted with the falsehoods of any contagious superstition" (*Inscriptiones latinae selectae*, 705).

---

[35] Cf. J. Jouanna, *Hippocrate: Les vents—De l'art* (Paris: Les Belles Lettres, 1988), 139, who exaggerates somewhat, for the Aristotelian *Problems* shows that "scientists" were capable of positing in a disease like leprosy or scabies a direct transmission of infective material without invoking an aerial intermediary.

[36] Mme. Marie-Hélène Congourdeau kindly drew my attention to a Greek Christian parallel: Epiphanius of Cyprus, *Panarion* VII.25, claimed that the Nicolaitans were afflicted by heresy as "bodies are corrupted by other bodies through ἐγκεντρισμός (a sting?), scabies, and leprosy".

In all this it is perhaps foolish to seek to distinguish between degrees of propriety in the application of a metaphor, or to differentiate medical from non-medical. Many of those who talked of the contagion of illness or of heresy would not have been able to explain in what way they thought that the "common touch" worked, and few, if any, would have restricted the touch to the mere physical person-to-person transmission of a noxious substance. What mattered was the consequence, the "sharing" of the disease, rather than the action of touching itself. Yet, although in almost every instance, *contagio* bears the negative implication that the touch brings with it something harmful, this connotation was often strengthened by the use of verbs such as "pollute", "contaminate", "stain", or "defile", each of which, to a modern observer, involves a different metaphorical mechanism. To decide between primary and secondary meanings in such a conjunction of metaphor is impossible, and one can do little more than emphasize the general field of meaning that is inhabited by both or all these metaphors.[37]

Sheep and goats

One final problem remains to be tackled. The evidence assembled by Marx proves beyond any doubt that many Greek authors, expressly or implicitly, believed that some diseases could be passed, directly or indirectly, from person to person, and that proximity to the sick was extremely dangerous. An even greater abundance of examples can be culled from modern Latin dictionaries, so much so that one may suspect that by AD 300 *contagio* had become a dead metaphor or at least one that no longer carried any implication about the precise mode of disease transmission.[38] Yet one group of authors is conspicuously absent from Marx's list—the medical writers, a fact that has often triggered speculation and talk of a contrast between medical and non-medical views of transmission. The percipience of Thucydides, the historian and victim of the plague of Athens, is set against the apparent silence of the Hippocratic Cor-

[37] L. Bodson, "Le vocabulaire latin des maladies pestilentielles et épizootiques," in G. Sabbah, ed., *Le latin médical*, 216–41, at 226, cites the collocation in glossaries of the words *contagio* and *coinquinatio*, and the use together of the same words by veterinary writers.

[38] Cf. the splendidly rhetorical passage in Cyprian, *De mortalitate* 8, where the sufferings of the sick are listed; they include those whose "feet and limbs are being amputated by the contagion of morbid putrefaction"; cf. 16: Enoch deserved his translation "from the contagion of this world".

pus, his understanding of the perils of proximity against a blind belief in the workings of bad air.[39]

One explanation for the non-appearance of discussions of the principle of contagion in medical authors can be quickly discounted. The sheer abundance of the non-medical evidence, the frequency of the metaphor in Latin, and the testimony of such late authors as Theodore Priscian and Caelius Aurelianus are enough to exclude the possibility that this was a theory unknown to doctors. Plutarch's dinner guests were familiar with medical and scientific writings, and were occasionally joined by doctors: even if the actual conversations were stylized inventions, their context, of an easy interchange between medical and non-medical men, was not. Besides, as we shall see, veterinary writers were familiar with the idea of diseases of proximity, and with segregation as a remedy. Galen, so often derided for his neglect of contagion, shows himself well aware of the phenomenon when in his story of the sufferer from leprosy who was unexpectedly cured by the effects of viper flesh he remarked that some of those who had previously associated with the man had themselves shared his disease.[40]

A variant of this explanation for the absence of any strictly medical discussion of contagion would emphasize the very fragility of our information on ancient medicine. Much of what survives represents one tradition, that of Hippocratic medicine as defined and mediated by Galen and the Galenists. Alternative theories, for example those of the Empiricists, Asclepiades, and the Methodists, are invoked only to make up for the deficiencies of the Hippocratics, e.g. in gynaecology, or are presented by Galen and his followers in a hostile and misleading manner. Even where verbatim quotations from Erasistratus or Asclepiades survive, they are frequently given without the context that would assist a proper interpretation. The Latin translators and compilers of the fourth century and later are concerned more with practical therapies than with theoretical debates, conscious of the need for brevity in a society increasingly lacking in scholarly aids.

---

[39] Cf. Holladay and Poole, "Thucydides and the Plague of Athens." The weakness of their argument for a Thucydidean *understanding* of contagion is pointed out by J. Solomon, "Thucydides and the Recognition of Contagion," *Maia* 37 (1985): 121–2, and by J. N. Longrigg, "Epidemic, Ideas and Classical Athenian Society," in *Epidemics and Ideas: Essays on the Historical Perception of Pestilence*, ed. Terence Ranger and Paul Slack (Cambridge: Cambridge University Press, 1992), 21–44, esp. 33–5.

[40] Galen, *Subfig. emp.* X; ed. Deichgräber, 75; *De simp. med.* XI.1: Kühn, XII, 312.

This argument is not without force, especially as medical historians tend unthinkingly to equate the medical texts that have survived with medical ideas in general. It is salutary to be reminded just how much has disappeared, and how much our knowledge of past debates comes only from the winning side. But the importance of the vagaries of transmission should not be exaggerated here, for, as we have seen, *contagio* is scarcely mentioned in the large Methodist compendium of Caelius Aurelianus, and not at all in the much earlier *On Medicine* by Cornelius Celsus, whose summaries of the views of the medical sects combine fairness with independence. Nor is the Hippocratic Corpus the monolith often imagined; indeed, recent scholars have stressed the variety of debates and ideas revealed within its numerous treatises. While the Greek compendia of Late Antiquity become increasingly Galenist in orientation, their Latin counterparts are far more open to other views than those of the Hippocratics or Dogmatists. Besides, it is clear from hints in Galen that he was aware of arguments that could have involved contagion and were similar to those reported by Plutarch.[41] Thus even if it is admitted that some medical texts in the Hippocratic Corpus may have been written before a theory of contagion became well known, that some authors may never have come across such a doctrine in their education and reading, and that, in general, Greek authors emphasized the sharing and the pollution of the disease and Latin the contact, enough remains to suggest that the marginality of contagion theory in our medical sources, and particularly the Greek, was not entirely the result of benign neglect, ignorance, or linguistic fashion. Nor is it fair to assume that medical authors rejected theories obvious to the general public out of prejudice and a devotion to outmoded theory.

One part of the explanation for the non-appearance of contagion theory in medical texts may lie in the fact that it appeared to require a mechanistic view of the universe and man. Such a standpoint was acceptable to Epicureans and Democritean philosophers, but anathema to Platonists, Aristotelians, and doctors, who, in general, favoured a vitalist approach or who, like the Empiricists, refused to investigate causation. Since Galen in particular was strongly opposed to Epicureanism and to Methodism, it is hardly surprising that in the tradition that he shaped there is little mention of this concept. But as we have seen, Galen is not the only medical writer to survive, nor Hippocratism the only theory to be recorded.

---

[41] Nutton, "The Seeds of Disease," 1–9.

A second reason may simply be that the great killer infectious diseases were absent for long periods from the Mediterranean world in Antiquity. Pandemics appear only rarely—perhaps the Athenian plague of 430–27, the "Antonine plague" (probably smallpox) that ravaged the Roman world in the 160s, a plague in North Africa in the mid-third century, and, in the mid-sixth century, the plague of Justinian (probably the first instance of bubonic plague)—and epidemics are recorded only for particular areas and seldom lasted long.[42] Even if it is admitted that such words for plague as *loimos*, *lues*, *pestis*, and *pestilentia* might hide a multitude of different modern diseases, the small range of diseases recorded in our sources as spread by "contagion" is striking.[43] Neither in literature nor in medicine do we find expressions of horror at occurrences, and, still more, recurrences, of epidemics like bubonic plague, typhus, typhoid, measles, or cholera, familiar from medieval or modern periods. In our state of ignorance of the epidemiology of the ancient world, it would be foolish to claim that epidemic diseases were less studied because there were fewer epidemics, but a relatively stable disease environment may well have played its part in concentrating the attention of medical writers on the diseases of individuals rather than groups.

A third reason has to do with the context in which "contagious diseases" were observed. It is striking that Thucydides in describing how victims died in the plague of Athens expressly compares them to sheep, as they became "filled" with the disease through treating one another.[44] The same comparison is found in other reports of pestilence by historians, as well as in the

[42] R. Sallares, *The Ecology of the Ancient Greek World* (London: Duckworth, 1991), 221–93; R. P. Duncan-Jones, "The Impact of the Antonine Plague," *Journal of Roman Archaeology* 9 (1996): 108–36. If "the bubonic plague" mentioned by Rufus as ravaging Libya, Egypt, and Syria around 60 BC is identical with modern bubonic plague, and was endemic in that region for much longer, it is odd that there is no major pandemic recorded before the plague of Justinian. Other identifications of the plague of buboes are perhaps to be preferred. See also J. N. Biraben, *Les hommes et la peste* (Paris: Mouton, 1975–6).

[43] Cf. Marx, *Origines contagii*, 137–41, for the list of ancient disease names, some of which can be referred to the same modern condition.

[44] Thucydides, *Hist.* II.lii.4. His "dying like [the] sheep", a phrase as common in Greek as in English, does not imply, as some have thought, that Athenian sheep also died of the plague—they had in fact been removed far away from the city. Nor need we agree with a later (Byzantine) commentator that Thucydides meant that sheep "are receptive to and capable of sharing the disease". But the more the simile is regarded as a cliché, the stronger the case for claiming that such frequent and numerous deaths were easiest observed in flocks and herds.

celebrated description of plague in Virgil's *Georgics* III.[45] Earlier, in his first *Eclogue*, I.50, Virgil had warned of the harm that a sick animal could cause to its neighbours in the flock. The same insights can be found in the first-century writer on agriculture, Columella, and, still more, in the fourth- or fifth-century works on veterinary medicine by Vegetius and the pseudonymous Chiron. They all emphasize how the presence of a single diseased animal can quickly infect a whole flock or herd; the disease passes quickly from one beast to another, contaminates, befouls (*coinquinat*), and destroys one's animals. Scab, glanders, "elephantiasis", and "pestilence" can all ravage in this way, and the more animals herded together, the more terrible the mortality. Vigilance and care are continually required of the herdsman, for a single loose animal can bring back a whole array of disease and destroy its fellows. These ideas can be found also in the Greek veterinary corpus, for Apsyrtus (fl. AD 320) remarked on the spread of glanders and "elephantiasis" through proximity.[46]

But not all veterinary writers share this concern with contagion. There is no mention of contagion in the Latin writer Pelagonius, familiar though he was with texts that discussed it; and the excerptors of the various collections of horse-medicine, when they presented snippets of medical theory alongside their lists of remedies, seem to have omitted discussions of aetiology that involved proximity. Even though Apsyrtus' views on the origins of glanders are noted in the Berlin collection, those in Paris and Lyons make no mention of it, and an author like Theomnestus, who expressly refers to Apsyrtus, does not appear to follow either his aetiology or his therapeutics.[47] In short, although some veterinary authors talk about contagion in some detail, others, whether deliberately or through accidental loss in the process of later excerpting, say nothing at all about it.

It is in veterinary medicine that one can see most clearly the strengths and weaknesses of the ancient theories of contagion. One can appreciate the soundness of the observation that links the spread of a disease like glanders to

[45] Cf. David West, "Two Plagues: Virgil, *Georgics* 3, 478–566 and Lucretius 6, 1090–1286," in *Creative Imitation and Latin Poetry*, ed. D. West and A. Woodman (Cambridge: Cambridge University Press, 1979), 71–88, 221–2.

[46] These examples are discussed by Bodson, "Le vocabulaire latin des maladies pestilentielles et épizootiques."

[47] *Hippiatrica berolinensia*, Chaps. ii–iii. Cf. K. D. Fischer, "Genera huius morbi maleos numero VII. Eine Infekionskrankheit (Malleus) und ihre Unterarten im Spiegel des antiken veterinärmedizinischen Schrifttums," in G. Sabbah, ed., *Le latin médical*, 351–65.

proximity—and the wisdom of a recommendation to segregate infected animals, and remove the healthy to pasture as far away as possible.[48] As advice, it is akin to what Cornelius Celsus had earlier recommended for humans: in time of pestilence travel or an overseas trip was the best preventative medicine (*On Medicine* I.x.1). Both Columella and Vegetius think of contagion in terms of the transfer of foetid breath (*halitus* or *odor*) between animals, but this is only one way in which they consider that glanders, for instance, arises. General climatic conditions can change the surrounding air so that it becomes pestiferous, or there can be, either in consequence, in addition, or independently, harmful alteration (*corruptio*) in the blood or the breath of the individual animal. Scab, a disease considered contagious by Columella and Vegetius, is ascribed by Theomnestus (*Hipp. berol.* LXIX.16) only to the corruption of the humours and blood as a result of heat. The standard explanation for the various forms of *malis*, glanders, emphasizes internal changes within the animal as much as any general atmospheric change, and certainly far more than any contact with an infected animal.

Thus, even among those who most often refer to diseases of proximity or contiguity, the veterinarians, *contagio* is only one of several explanations for the appearance of disease in an individual. Far more often they use the categories of internal bodily change (in humours, elements, atoms, or other substances) and external, general alteration in the surrounding air. This is not to say that they were unaware that, in certain conditions, proximity to the diseased animal was itself dangerous; rather that the way in which the danger was explained did not necessarily or only involve contiguity. Besides, the number of human diseases in which direct touch, *contagio* in the most literal sense of the word, was invoked was very small, leprosy, rabies, and scabies, since in most "contagious" conditions the sufferer reputedly exhaled a foetid, poisonous, or noxious "miasma" into the air. Even so, the presence of a polluting miasma did not guarantee that others would become infected: that depended also on individual susceptibility, on the make-up of the individual body. Veterinarians, as well as doctors, stressed the need to prevent the arrival of disease in an individual patient, human or animal, by securing in advance the best possible state of health in order to defy the potentially dangerous external attack by a miasma. If the same diseased condition could be also produced from internal causes, then there was all the more reason to build up the body's internal defences. In practical terms, therefore, a theory of

[48] Apsyrtus, *Hippiatrica berolinensia* ii.9, iii.1.

contagion, even among those who spoke in terms of *contagio*, was of restricted value.

There was another reason why human doctors should concern themselves little with contiguity as an element in aetiology or therapy. Veterinarians could recommend the removal, segregation, even slaughter, of an affected animal. Such methods were not acceptable to human doctors. As Caelius Aurelianus put it (*Chron.* IV.13), one could lock up or exile sufferers from leprosy in an attempt to stop the spread of the disease—and this might have been done in certain cities—but the humanitarian ethic of medicine forbade it.[49] The doctor had an obligation to care, not to abandon. This ethic of a Methodist doctor was shared by others in the Hippocratic tradition. Both Galen and Aretaeus record the same story of a leper cured by drink from a jar into which a viper had fallen. Galen, in his elaborate way of storytelling, mentions the humanity and compassion of those who, despite their fears, and despite the evidence that the leper's associates had themselves caught the disease, nevertheless tried to help, if only by supplying what they thought was a fatal potion that would end his misery. Aretaeus more succinctly reports with apparent disapproval that "many have exiled into the mountains or desert even their closest friends".[50] In his subsequent description of the cure of the disease, which, in his view, is almost impossible once leprosy has taken hold, Aretaeus remarks that men fear to associate with lepers, just as with wild beasts: "for the infection (taint) is easily shared through breath".[51] Doctors like Caelius, Galen, and Aretaeus were thus aware of the dangers of contiguity in certain diseases, and of the preventative measures that some might think necessary, but they were also prepared to condemn them as inhuman.

By far the strongest reason for the apparent neglect by ancient doctors of contagion theory lies in their social situation, in their inability to enforce the

[49] This passage is not noted in O. Temkin, *Hippocrates in a World of Pagans and Christian* (Baltimore: Johns Hopkins University Press, 1991), or in Deichgräber, *Medicus gratiosus.* Expulsion of lepers from the community was not unknown (cf. Temkin, *Hippocrates*, 162), but I know of no evidence for imprisonment, although that is not impossible.

[50] For the Galenic references, see above, n. 40; for Aretaeus, *Signs chron. dis.* II.xiii.20: *CMG,* II, 90:7–22. For the relationship between these two accounts, see my "Style and Context in the Method of Healing," in *Galen's Method of Healing*, ed. F. Kudlien and R. J. Durling (Leiden: E. J. Brill, 1991), 1–25, at 11–13.

[51] Aretaeus, *Cur. chron. dis.* II.xiii.1: *CMG,* II, 168. The Greek metaphor *baphe* comes, like *infectio,* originally from dyeing. It is perhaps worth noting that recent studies of leprosy, Hansen's disease, suggest that it is not contagious, despite the belief of generations of doctors to the contrary.

consequences of that theory, exclusion and quarantine. However much they might be aware of the dangers of contiguity, their authority was hardly strong enough to break the bonds of family care for the sick. The sister of Thrasylochus in Isocrates' speech is condemned by the orator precisely because she failed in her family duty to tend the sick. Provincial governors and civic councils, although they might employ physicians to reside in the community, did not intervene in the doctor–patient relationship, and it is arguable whether any ancient city had developed the complex administration and the concentration of power and authority that enabled Italian cities from the fourteenth century onwards to impose expensive and draconian measures against the plague.[52] Even when, as Caelius Aurelianus implies, segregation was thought advisable, one should note the very different attitudes taken towards members of the community and those outside it. It is the non-citizen, the alien, who is to be removed, locked up, or worse; the citizen is recommended to depart, as if for a holiday, and there is no suggestion that leprosy will make the sufferer an unacceptable guest in the region to which he or she is sent. Even had ancient physicians been strong believers in contagion theory, it is very doubtful if they had the social power to compel others to go against the most sacred of moral duties, to care for one's kin and dependants.

Such a stark choice was, however, scarcely necessary. On almost all ancient schemata, contagion, whether in the strict sense of a disease transmitted by touch or in the wider one of a disease of contiguity, was only rarely invoked to explain the origin of an illness, and, even when it was, it formed only one part, and not necessarily the most important part, of a complex of overlapping alternatives. Both individual susceptibility and, often, the pollution of the ambient air were far more significant than transmissibility of the disease, and both could be more easily combated with the means at the disposal of the physician. Unlike contagion theory, neither involved as a consequence the isolation, or worse, of members of the family. The idea of a purely mechanistic transmission of disease from person to person was similarly hard to reconcile with theories that emphasized individuality as well as a vitalist view of the body. Given that none of the infective agents could be observed, let alone identified, until the nineteenth century, it is hardly surprising that the

[52] For civic doctors in Antiquity and the Italian Middle Ages, see my *From Democedes to Harvey*, Chapter VI. Carlo M. Cipolla, in a variety of short books, has explicated the Italian procedures against plague, especially in the sixteenth and seventeenth century, e.g. *Fighting the Plague in Seventeenth-Century Italy* (Madison: University of Wisconsin Press, 1981).

debate, if such there was, centred on metaphors, or that the process of disease-transmission was associated most often with the air, whose foulness could be perceived by smell and occasionally sight. Under such circumstances, it makes little sense to contrast, as some modern historians have done, rational medical explanations with the pre-rational, or irrational, miasmatic explanations for sin and religious pollution. Both occupied the same explanatory field, overlapped, and interchanged, and the presence of one metaphor did not of itself exclude what might seem today contradictory alternatives.

Finally, one cannot but insist strongly on the dangers of the false friend. Because words like *contagio* and *infectio* are etymologically related to modern English or French words with a specific medical meaning, there is a great danger that the modern understanding of the process of contagion and infection is to be traced back to antiquity simply on the basis of linguistics, or that the ancients are to be dismissed as unobservant or foolish for not talking in such terms. As we have seen, the discussion of contagion has been bedevilled, often unwittingly, by this linguistic confusion. This paper has tried to chart a way between the known and the unknown in an examination of the *Origines contagii*, between diseases of touch and diseases of proximity, between observations and explanations. If, in the end, it says little more than what a German doctoral student wrote over 150 years ago, that is in itself a tribute to the diligence and acumen of the other Karl Marx.[53]

[53] I am grateful for comments on this paper to the London audience, and especially to Karl-Heinz Leven and James Longrigg.

8

A Ninth-Century Muslim Scholar's Discussion of Contagion

Lawrence I. Conrad

It is well known that from an early point much of medieval Islamic scholarship adopted a negative attitude toward the doctrine of contagion. A tradition of the Prophet Muḥammad proclaimed *lā ʿadwā*, "No contagion", and henceforth Islam refused to credit the notion that a disease could be transmitted directly from an ill person to a healthy one.

Such is the conclusion often drawn in modern scholarship, but in fact the situation is not and has never been so simple. Three points in particular must be borne in mind from the outset. First, the Arabic term normally translated in English as "contagion", *ʿadwā*, is actually a term with a far broader meaning.[1] The root *ʿ–d–w* conveys the general idea of transitiveness, transference, the passage of something from one locus to another, or its situation with respect to them; various verbal and nominal forms derived from this root that convey the idea of transmission of disease therefore also have other transitive or relational connotations. Thus the form I and II verbs mean, *inter alia*, to leave something (i.e. to pass beyond it), to turn away, to misbehave or deviate (i.e. to exceed proper bounds or transgress), and to pounce upon something. The form IV verb has especially strong transitive meanings, such as to cause someone to do or feel something, to express a quality or

[1] See Ernst Seidel, "Die Lehre von der Kontagion bei den Arabern", *Archiv für Geschichte der Medizin* 6 (1913): 81–93; Manfred Ullmann, *Die Medizin im Islam* (Leiden: E. J. Brill, 1970), 242–50; *idem, Islamic Medicine* (Edinburgh: Edinburgh University Press, 1978), 86–96; Felix Klein-Franke, *Vorlesungen über die Medizin im Islam* (Wiesbaden: Franz Steiner Verlag, 1982), 17–19; Muḥammad ʿAlī al-Bār, *Al-ʿAdwā: bayna l-ṭibb wa-ḥadīth al-muṣṭafā*, 4th ed. (Jedda: al-Dār al-saʿūdīya li-l-nashr wa-l-tawzīʿ, 1401/1981), 23–70.

trait of character to someone else, and to assist, support, or avenge someone.[2]

The broad transitive sense of the root *ʿ–d–w* brings us to our second point. In medieval Arabic texts the term *ʿadwā* is used in the sense of "transmissibility", and hence encompasses the modern notions of both contagion and infection. Quite often it is clearly the former sense which is meant, as in sayings like: "No sick one conveys illness to a healthy one." But in fact, there was never any attempt to draw a sharp distinction between the two. Hence, although in some of the cases to be considered here either the one sense or the other is clearly more appropriate, it must be borne in mind that the modern epidemiological distinctions between infection and contagion were unknown in the medieval Middle East, or indeed, as the studies in this volume demonstrate, anywhere else in the world until early modern times.

Finally, it must be recognized that there is no single "Islamic" position on contagion. The debate over *ʿadwā* began in early Islamic times and is still discussed today among Muslim physicians committed both to their faith and to their professions as modern medics. By focusing on one of the central contributions, it will hopefully be possible to convey some sense of the main issues under discussion and how medical matters were and in some senses continue to be enmeshed in other considerations important in Islamic societies.

The author of concern to us here is Ibn Qutayba (d. 276/889), one of the most important literary figures of the ninth-century Middle East. Born in al-Kūfa (but usually associated with al-Baṣra), Ibn Qutayba was a scholar of very broad education and studied with some of the greatest authorities of his day. He had close connections with the ruling ʿAbbāsid house in Baghdad and served for a time as judge of Dīnawar. His literary output was prodigious and indicative of the talents of the many-faceted scholars of the period. He wrote a historical digest that is still a useful source today, a compendium on poets that begins with an important analysis of Arabic poetry, works on obscure and problematic terms and passages in the Qur'ān and *ḥadīth* (reports of the deeds, sayings, and opinions of the Prophet Muḥammad and other early Muslims), a manual for use by government secretaries in need of a well-rounded education, a question-and-answer text on religio-theological

[2] See, for example, Ibn Manẓūr (d. 711/1311), *Lisān al-ʿarab* (Beirut: Dār Ṣādir, 1374–6/1955–6), XV, 31b:7–43b:10; Murtaḍā al-Zabīdī (d. 1205/1791), *Tāj al-ʿarūs* (Cairo: al-Maṭbaʿa al-khayrīya, AH 1306–8), X, 235:12–238:33.

problems, a compendium of literary pieces on a wide range of topics, and much more besides.[3]

The background to Ibn Qutayba's discussion of contagion extends back to pre-Islamic Arabia, where the Arab tribes considered that epidemics were caused by demons and other spirit beings who spread pestilence among mankind by means of their various weapons.[4] They also considered it obvious that such maladies were likewise transmissible. In the sense in which the pre-Islamic Arabs understood the term, contagion was seen most clearly in the spread of disease among their herds, the most frequently cited example being mange in camels. A frequently cited example of this is the verse of Dhu'ayb ibn Ka'b, describing how undeserved calamity is sometimes visited upon the innocent:

> The one who has harmed you and with your foe sides
> Is the one who should suffer the force of your blow.
> But sometimes the camels with mange on their hides
> Will infect the healthy and thus lay them low.[5]

---

[3]The authoritative work on Ibn Qutayba remains Gérard Lecomte, *Ibn Qutayba (mort en 276/889): l'homme, son oeuvre, ses idées* (Damascus: Institut français de Damas, 1965). See also Lecomte's article on Ibn Qutayba in the *Encyclopaedia of Islam*, New Edition, ed. H. A. R. Gibb *et al.* (Leiden: E. J. Brill, 1960–proceeding), III, 844b–847b.

[4]See Ḥassān ibn Thābit (d. *ca.* 40/659), *Dīwān*, ed. Walid N. 'Arafat (Leiden: E. J. Brill, 1971), II, 172:10–13; al-Jāḥiẓ (d. 255/868), *Kitāb al-ḥayawān*, ed. 'Abd al-Salām Muḥammad Hārūn, 2nd ed. (Cairo: Muṣṭafā al-Bābī al-Ḥalabī, 1385–8/1965–9), I, 351:5–9; VI, 218:12–220:8; Ibn Qutayba, *'Uyūn al-akhbār*, ed. Aḥmad Zakī al-'Adawī (Cairo: Dār al-kutub al-miṣrīya, 1343–8/1925–30), II, 114:6; al-Mas'ūdī (d. 345/956), *Murūj al-dhahab*, ed. Charles Pellat (Beirut: Université libanaise, 1966–79), III, 214:8–12; al-Tha'ālibī (d. 429/1038), *Thimār al-qulūb*, ed. Muḥammad Abū l-Faḍl Ibrāhīm (Cairo: Dār nahḍat Miṣr, 1384/1965), 68:1–69:2; Ibn Abī l-Ḥadīd (d. 656/1258), *Sharḥ nahj al-balāgha*, ed. Muḥammad Abū l-Faḍl Ibrāhīm (Cairo: 'Īsā al-Bābī al-Ḥalabī, 1959–64), XV, 240:2–8.

[5]Abū 'Ubayda (d. 207/822), *Naqā'iḍ Jarīr wa-l-Farazdaq*, ed. A. A. Bevan (Leiden: E. J. Brill, 1905–12), II, 1026:3; Ibn 'Abd Rabbih (d. 328/940), *Al-'Iqd al-farīd*, ed. Aḥmad Amīn, Aḥmad al-Zayn, and Ibrāhīm al-Abyārī (Cairo: Lajnat al-ta'līf wa-l-tarjama wa-l-nashr, 1363–70/1944–56), V, 237:6. For other examples, see al-Mufaḍḍal al-Ḍabbī (d. *ca.* 170/786), *Dīwān al-mufaḍḍalīyāt*, ed. Charles James Lyall (Oxford: Clarendon Press, 1921), 752:7–11; al-Ḥumaydī (d. 219/834), *Al-Musnad*, ed. Ḥabīb al-Raḥmān al-A'ẓamī (Hyderabad: Dā'irat al-ma'ārif al-'uthmānīya, AH 1381–2), II, 308:9–309:3 no. 705; al-Bukhārī (d. 256/870), *Al-Jāmi' al-ṣaḥīḥ*, ed. Ludolf Krehl and T. W. Juynboll (Leiden: E. J. Brill, 1862–1908), II, 16pu–17:4 *Buyū'* no. 36; Abū l-Faraj al-Iṣfahānī (d. 356/967), *Kitāb al-aghānī*, ed. Naṣr al-Hūrīnī (Cairo: al-Maṭba'a al-kubrā al-amīrīya, AH 1284–5), IV, 155:26–7.

An anonymous poet refers to how the destruction of warfare overwhelms even those who seek to avoid involvement, just as mange spreads from sick to healthy camels:

> War extends its grasping hand
> And shows the innocent no respect,
> Like healthy camels in a land
> That nearby mangy ones infect.[6]

That *'adwā* was perceived in a far broader sense than is comprehended by the modern notion of contagion has already been stressed above. But the point is highlighted by several traditions bearing on the interpretation of a passage in the Qur'ān in Sūrat al-Nūr (24), vs. 61: "There is no fault in the blind, and there is no fault in the lame, and there is no fault in the sick. . . ."[7] Early traditions explaining this verse assert that until its revelation "people were on their guard against the blind, the lame, and the sick",[8] thus suggesting that not only diseases, but also physical disabilities, were feared for the possibility that they might be transmitted to healthy individuals.

Muslims in early Islamic times seem to have considered it perfectly acceptable to continue to speak of disease in terms of these traditional ideas, and even in traditions cited as the words of the Prophet these perceptions still appear. A famous tradition has it, for example, that Muḥammad advised: "Flee from the leper as you would flee from a lion",[9] and others claim that he refused to receive lepers[10] and advised people not to allow their gaze to linger on them.[11] But as Islam developed as a spiritual system, the old notions concerning contagion could not remain unopposed. First and foremost, in a religious order dominated by the doctrine of an all-powerful and all-ordaining God, there was no place for the concession of devastating powers to minor spirits, or

[6] Abū Tammām (d. 231/845), *Dīwān al-ḥamāsa*, ed. with the commentary of al-Tibrīzī (d. 502/1109) by Muḥammad 'Abd al-Qādir Sa'īd al-Rāfi'ī (Beirut: Dār al-qalam, n.d.), I, 154:4.

[7] See A. J. Arberry, *The Koran Interpreted* (Oxford: Oxford University Press, 1964), 360.

[8] Ibn Abī Shayba (d. 235/849), *Al-Muṣannaf fī l-ḥadīth wa-l-āthār*, ed. Mukhtār Aḥmad al-Nadawī (Bombay: al-Dār al-salafiya, 1399–1403/1979–83), VIII, 130:10–13.

[9] See, for example, 'Abd al-Razzāq al-Ṣan'ānī (d. 211/827), *Muṣannaf*, ed. Ḥabīb al-Raḥmān al-A'ẓamī (Beirut: al-Maktab al-islāmī, 1390–2/1970–2), X, 405:5–6; XI, 204:12–205:1; Ibn Abī Shayba, *Muṣannaf*, VIII, 132:3–5; IX, 44:5–7.

[10] Ibn Abī Shayba, *Muṣannaf*, VIII, 131ult–132:2; IX, 43pu–44:1.

[11] Al-Ṭayālisī (d. 204/819), *Musnad* (Hyderabad: Dā'irat al-ma'ārif al-niẓāmīya, AH 1321), 339:26–7 no. 2601; Ibn Abī Shayba, *Muṣannaf*, VIII, 132:6–8; IX, 44:2–4.

for a conception of disease causation that allowed for the capricious infection of one individual after another regardless of their good or evil deeds. As for "contagion", this notion was particularly prominent since it arose not only in connection with epidemic disease, but also with reference to leprosy.[12] From both of these concerns, there emerged a tradition of the Prophet in which Muḥammad says: *lā 'adwā*, "No contagion". That this denial of "contagion" was based on considerations far beyond those of medicine or the explanation of disease transmission is proven by the fact that this pronouncement usually occurs in a list of traditional beliefs now repudiated by Islam as baseless superstition: "No contagion, no omens from birds, no owl, no serpent". The "omens from birds" (*ṭiyara*) refers to the old augury custom of foretelling the future from the cries, flight, and alighting places of birds; the term for this was eventually generalized to cover all physical phenomena believed to influence or indicate the course of future events. The meaning of the "owl" (*hāma*) was disputed, but was believed in some circles to represent the spirit of a wrongfully slain man; it would never rest until his death had been properly avenged by the killing of his murderer. The "serpent" (*ṣafar*), also disputed, was regarded by some as a parasite that attacked and afflicted men in their bellies, and was considered more easily transmissible from one person to another than mange spreading among camels. All of these—"contagion", the omens from birds, the wandering owl, and the abdominal "serpent"—are repudiated because they are regarded as major constituent elements in a system of causation, based largely on concepts of pagan animism and simple caprice, which implies that crucial events in human life can be affected or directed by forces independent of and even contrary to the will of God. Viewed from the strictly monotheistic perspective of emergent Islam, in other words, there can be no contagion—in the sense in which it was understood at that time—because all things come from God.[13]

Other traditions arose to counter early pro-contagion views, but the response to the denial of "contagion" was the obvious one: does not simple

---

[12]See Michael W. Dols, "The Leper in Medieval Islamic Society," *Speculum* 58 (1983): 891–916.

[13]For some early examples of such statements, see Mālik ibn Anas (d. 179/795), *Al-Muwaṭṭa'*, ed. Muḥammad Fu'ād 'Abd al-Bāqī (Cairo: 'Īsā al-Bābī al-Ḥalabī, 1370/1951), II, 946:4–6 *'Ayn* no. 18; 'Abd Allāh ibn Wahb (d. 197/813), *Kitāb al-jāmi'*, ed. J. David-Weill (Cairo: Institut français d'archéologie orientale, 1939–48), I, 90:11–93ult; al-Ṭayālisī, *Musnad*, 265:2–3 no. 1961; 'Abd al-Razzāq, *Muṣannaf*, X, 404:15–405:3, 405:12–406:3; XI, 205:5–7; al-Ḥumaydī, *Musnad*, II, 308:9–309:3 no. 705.

manifest experience demonstrate that some diseases are indeed transmissible, and very quickly and easily so? The anti-contagionist camp had an answer in the form of a parable. The Prophet says, "No contagion", and a bedouin replies: "O Apostle of God, what about my camels? They are like gazelle does on the sand;[14] but let a mangy camel come and mix with them, and soon they are all mangy." The Prophet counters: "And who caused the mange in the first one?"[15] The answer is of course God. Similar traditions against contagion arose, and the result was that by the advent of the third/ninth century there were in circulation a broad range of sharply contradictory traditions on this subject and of course many others where, as with contagion, an old belief or custom was at first accepted in Islamic society and then rejected. These cases of contradiction also called into question the validity of the *ḥadīth* literature in general, both as a foundation for elaboration of law and as a model for proper pious conduct, since if the methods and materials of this field of inquiry were sound there ought not to be major contradictions within it. The rationalist theologians known as the Muʿtazila[16] were particularly stern in their critique of *ḥadīth*, and one of them, the Baṣran theologian al-Naẓẓām (d. *ca.* 230/845),[17] chose precisely the traditions on contagion to show that the scholars of *ḥadīth* had no coherent methodology for arriving at sound religious knowledge and that their materials were irredeemably flawed:

> How can it be [said] that they commit no errors, tell no lies, display no ignorance, and do not contradict one another, when those of them who relate from the Prophet—may the blessing and peace of God be upon him—that he said: "No contagion and no omens from birds in Islam", and that he also said: "And who infected the first one", are the [same] ones who relate that he said: "Flee from the leper as you would flee from a lion"; and

[14] I.e., their unblemished hides are like the tawny pelts of gazelles, which camouflage them against the background of the steppe.

[15] ʿAbd Allāh ibn Wahb, *Jāmiʿ*, I, 91:8–10; Aḥmad ibn Ḥanbal (d. 242/855), *Musnad* (Cairo: al-Maṭbaʿa al-kubrā al-amīrīya, AH 1311), I, 269:14–17, 328:11–13, 440:24–9; II, 24pu–25:2, 267:2–5, 317:26–30; al-Bukhārī, *Ṣaḥīḥ*, IV, 57:6–11, 69:10–70:6, *Ṭibb* nos. 25, 53–4; Muslim (d. 261/874), *Ṣaḥīḥ*, ed. Muḥammad Fuʾād ʿAbd al-Bāqī (Cairo: ʿĪsā al-Bābī al-Ḥalabī, 1375–6/1955–6), IV, 1742:10–1743:6, *Salām* nos. 101–2

[16] *Encyclopaedia of Islam*, VII, 783a–793b.

[17] On al-Naẓẓām, see Josef van Ess, *Theologie und Gesellschaft im 2. und 3. Jahrhundert Hidschra. Eine Geschichte des religiösen Denkens im frühen Islam* (Berlin: Walter de Gruyter, 1991–5), III, 296–445, and for his views on knowledge and epistemology, 380–402.

> that a leper came to him to pledge his loyalty as a Muslim to him, but [the Prophet] sent him someone to take his pledge and did not allow him to come close to him, out of fear of being infected by him?[18]

As can be seen here, the issue is not so much medical problems of disease as the broader difficulties posed in other ways by the old materials on this subject. As it became entangled in questions of this kind, the issue of contagion became a symbol of the dispute over the legitimacy of various intellectual disciplines within emergent Islamic scholarship, and what the future of the various alternatives would or should be.

This brings us to Ibn Qutayba, who took up the challenge of al-Naẓẓām in his *Ta'wīl mukhtalif al-ḥadīth* ("Exegesis of Contradictory Traditions"), a book which represents the work of his mature years and was completed shortly after 256/870.[19] When his attention turns to contagion he has a circle of hypothetical antagonists—the Mu'tazila are certainly those meant here—challenge him with the discrepant traditions mentioned above: "This is all contradictory", the critics conclude, "with no common ground between the various views".[20]

Ibn Qutayba objects and asserts that in fact there is no contradiction at all. Invoking the doctrine of miasma (though he does not use this word) and a proposal for a distinction between "contagion" as a scientific concept and "contagion" as perceived in popular superstition, he argues that each interpretation has its context of time and place, and that if it is situated within its proper context the apparent contradictions disappear:

> Contagion is of two types, one of these being the contagion of leprosy. The leper gives off an odour so strong that it causes anyone who long remains in his presence or eats with him to fall ill. Similar is the case of the woman who is under a leper and has sexual intercourse with him in the same bedding; the affliction will be brought into contact with her, and she too may contract

---

[18] Josef van Ess, "Ein unbekanntes Fragment des Naẓẓām", in Wilhelm Hoenerbach, ed., *Der Orient in der Forschung: Festschrift für Otto Spies* (Wiesbaden: Otto Harrassowitz, 1967), 172.

[19] See Lecomte, *Ibn Qutayba*, 85–92. The text was translated by Lecomte in his *Le traité des divergences du Ḥadīṯ d'Ibn Qutayba* (Damascus: Institut français de Damas, 1962), with the passage on contagion at 114–16.

[20] Ibn Qutayba, *Ta'wīl mukhtalif al-ḥadīth*, ed. Muḥammad Muḥyī l-Dīn al-Aṣfar (Beirut: al-Maktab al-islāmī and Dār al-ishrāq, 1409/1989), 117ult.

> leprosy. The same applies to his children, who on many occasions come into contact with him. Such also are the cases of those suffering from consumption (*sull*), hectic fever (*daqq*), or purulent mange (*naqb*). When the physicians prescribe that one should not associate with a consumptive or a leper, they do not thereby imply a principle of contagion, but rather only have in mind the change in odour, which may well cause the one who smells it for an extended period to fall ill—physicians would be the last people to lend any credence to felicitous or evil omens.[21]

He then turns to the specific example of mange in camels, as discussed in Prophetic tradition:

> Similar is the case when the *nuqba*, a purulent mange, breaks out on a camel. When the others [in the herd] mix and intermingle with it and betake themselves to the same place where it kneels down to rest, they will be brought into contact with the fluid and pus issuing from it[s sores] and so contract the same disease from which it suffers. This is the principle of which the Apostle of God spoke: "Do not water the sick with the healthy." He was opposed to a diseased camel mingling with a healthy one, as the former's pus and rubbing[22] would expose the latter to the same disease.

Ibn Qutayba's next comments reveal that he was not the first one to attempt a rational harmonization of the contradictory traditions relevant to contagion:

> One circle of opinion holds the view that by prohibiting such mixing the Prophet wanted to keep people from falling into the sin of supposing that what has stricken their camels has come [to them] from the diseased ones. But so far as I am concerned there is no basis for this opinion, since we find manifest empirical evidence for the position set forth above.[23]

One representative of this view half a century prior to Ibn Qutayba was Abū 'Ubayd al-Qāsim ibn Sallām al-Harawī (d. 224/838), a native of Herat and a

[21] Ibid., 118:3–13.
[22] I.e. against another animal to relieve the itching of its sores.
[23] Ibid., 118:14–119:3.

widely travelled scholar primarily associated with Iraqi centres of learning.[24] Ibn Ḥajar al-ʿAsqalānī (d. 852/1449) several times cites him (without identifying the book he is using) for his negative comments on the continuing influence of old interpretations of the tradition disapproving the mixing of healthy with diseased animals:

> Some people attribute the tradition to fear of how that malady would affect the healthy animals, but this is the worst opinion that could be advocated on the *ḥadīth*, since it legitimates the superstitious interpretation that the tradition was meant to prohibit.

Abū ʿUbayd argues that the prohibition to the effect that one ought not to mix diseased camels with healthy ones was not declared by the Prophet in order to confirm the existence of contagion. Rather, what Muḥammad had in mind was a situation in which someone has healthy animals that fall ill by the decree of God; it might occur to the owner that this was a result of contagion, and thus lead him astray into religious misgivings and doubts.[25] It is likely that it is Abū ʿUbayd's view that Ibn Qutayba had in mind in his critical comments. Abū ʿUbayd was active in the same centres where Ibn Qutayba would later also move, and was simply too important and too well known for his work to escape the attention of such a very widely read scholar interested in similar subjects 50 years later.

Ibn Qutayba then proceeds to explain the second type of contagion he has in mind:

> The other type of contagion is the plague, which descends upon a land and causes [its inhabitants] to leave it out of fear of contagion. Sahl ibn Muḥammad told me that al-Aṣmaʿī told him, concerning one of the Basrans, that he fled from the plague, rode

[24] See Hans Gottschalk, "Abū ʿUbaid al-Qāsim b. Sallām," *Der Islam* 23 (1936): 264–83; Wilferd Madelung, "Early Sunnī Doctrine Concerning Faith as Reflected in the *Kitāb al-īmān* of Abū ʿUbayd al-Qāsim b. Sallām (d. 224/839)," *Studia Islamica* 32 (1970): 233–54.

[25] Cited in Ibn Ḥajar, *Badhl al-māʿūn fī faḍl al-ṭāʿūn*, ed. Aḥmad ʿIṣām ʿAbd al-Qādir (Riyadh: Dār al-ʿāṣima, AH 1411), 301:5–12; *idem*, *Fatḥ al-bārī bi-sharḥ Ṣaḥīḥ al-Bukhārī*, ed. ʿAbd al-Raḥmān Muḥammad (Cairo: al-Maṭbaʿa al-bahīya al-miṣrīya, AH 1348), X, 131:20–1.

off on a donkey, and headed with his family toward Safawān.[26] He heard a cameleer[27] singing behind him, saying:

By none will God be left behind
By clutching fast to a donkey's lead,
Nor from Him can one haven find
By turning to his dashing steed.
To each a fixed time God will bind
When he shall meet his death decreed.
The night-trod road may well but wind
To where God waits with writ to heed.[28]

The Apostle of God said: "If it is in the land in which you are, do not leave it." He also said: "If it is in a land, do not enter it." By the former he means: "Do not leave the land if the plague is there, as if you supposed that flight from the decree of God Almighty would save you from God himself." And by his saying "if the plague is in a land do not enter it", he means that your remaining in a place where there is no plague would provide you with greater peace of mind and more agreeable living con-

[26] A village and important watering place a day's journey south of al-Baṣra; see Yāqūt (d. 626/1229), *Mu'jam al-buldān*, ed. Ferdinand Wüstenfeld (Leipzig: F. A. Brockhaus, 1866–73), III, 98pu–99:2.

[27] I.e. a *ḥādī*, a herdsman who sings to camels in order to call them in from pasture or attract them to water before a long journey. See the poem cited in Kushājim (d. 360/971), *Dīwān*, ed. Khayrīya Muḥammad Maḥfūẓ (Baghdad: Wizārat al-i'lām, 1390/1970), 324:1–325:2 no. 303; *idem*, *Adab al-nadīm*, ed. Nabīl 'Aṭīya (Baghdad: Wizārat al-thaqāfa wa-l-i'lām, 1990), 56:1–8; Abū Ḥayyān al-Tawḥīdī (d. 414/1023), *Al-Baṣā'ir wa-l-dhakhā'ir*, ed. Wadād al-Qāḍī (Beirut: Dār Ṣādir, 1408/1988), II, 110:6–111:1. Cf. also Jibrail S. Jabbur, *The Bedouins and the Desert: Aspects of Nomadic Life in the Arab East*, trans. Lawrence I. Conrad (Albany: State University of New York Press, 1995), 230–2.

[28] For the various versions of this famous story, see al-Jāḥiẓ, *Ḥayawān*, III, 461:8–12, from al-Aṣma'ī (d. 213/828); *idem*, *Al-Bayān wa-l-tabyīn*, ed. 'Abd al-Salām Muḥammad Hārūn (Cairo: Lajnat al-ta'līf wa-l-tarjama wa-l-nashr, 1367–70/1948–50), III, 278:7–10; Ibn Qutayba, *'Uyūn al-akhbār*, I, 144:17–20, from al-Aṣma'ī.

> ditions....It is this sense of contagion of which the Apostle of God speaks when he says: "No contagion."[29]

There are some problems with this effort to resolve the problems put to traditionists by al-Naẓẓām. Belief in *'adwā* as a living willing force appears to have been a very old perspective, but one that the many references to "contagion" in pre-Islamic and early Islamic poetry and oral lore suggest had in time given way to a more naturalistic view. While there was no small element of superstition to traditional beliefs where disease was concerned, most Arab observers from the sixth century onward viewed the actual transmissibility of disease from one victim to another in practical terms, as a matter of simple empirical observation. Further, it is clear that the reason for the Islamic opposition to the doctrine of "contagion" was not so much that it amounted to pagan superstition—many aspects of ancient Arabian lore survived on into Islamic times—but that it was regarded as a diminution of the role of God as the author of all things. And it is quite unclear why Ibn Qutayba seeks to draw a distinction between *'adwā* as applied to leprosy and *'adwā* as applied to plague.

In other respects, however, his discussion is an accurate reflection of the social milieu that produced it. Earlier treatments of the subject had betrayed no trace of influence from medical thinking, for the simple reason that there was precious little formal humoral medicine anywhere in the domains of Islam until late in the second half of the eighth century.[30] Ibn Qutayba's material, on the other hand, comes from a time when formal physicians flourished in Baghdad, translations from Syriac and Greek were being produced at a rapid pace, and formal medical institutions (such as hospitals) were emerging. Hence his ability to comment on what physicians say about "contagion". It was, in fact, in the very next generation after Ibn Qutayba's death that the Syrian physician Qusṭā ibn Lūqā (d. *ca.* 300/912) devoted an essay to conta-

[29]Ibn Qutayba, *Ta'wīl mukhtalif al-ḥadīth,* 119:4–19. His argument is also repeated in full—unfortunately with many misreadings and omissions by a scribe or the modern editor—in al-Sharīf al-Murtaḍā (d. 436/1034), *Ghurar al-fawā'id wa-durar al-qalā'id* (= *Al-Amālī*), ed. Muḥammad Abū l-Faḍl Ibrāhīm (Cairo: 'Īsā al-Bābī al-Ḥalabī, 1373/1954), II, 200:10–202:12.

[30]This question is discussed in detail in Lawrence I. Conrad and Vivian Nutton, *Jundīshāpūr: From Myth to History* (Princeton: Darwin Press, forthcoming).

gion in which it was discussed and explained purely in medical/philosophical terms.[31]

Though his discussion in the *Taʾwīl mukhtalif al-ḥadīth* clearly seeks to vindicate the traditions of the Prophet, it is significant that, first, he does not argue against contagion as a valid medical doctrine, and second, as we have already seen above, that in the discussion by Abū ʿUbayd he already had an argument to hand that would explain away the contradictions among the contagion traditions, and yet decided to reject it. This suggests that while Ibn Qutayba was keen to protect *ḥadīth* from its critics, he did not want this effort to involve a repudiation of the doctrine of contagion.

Outside of the context of the problem of contradictions in Prophetic *ḥadīth* his true opinion on the subject of contagion is easier to discern. In the *ʿUyūn al-akhbār*, a work dedicated to a broad synthetic approach to culture incorporating material from many fields of intellectual endeavour, the subject of contagion arises again—if implicitly—in a brief discussion of leprosy. Here too Ibn Qutayba cites traditions from the Prophet about the disease, but only those that uphold a pro-contagion position. And added to these are other materials of a similar orientation. The Baṣran Qatāda ibn Diʿāma (d. 117/735) is cited for a report according to which a leper is driven away because it is thought that he has been cursed (*balaghanī annahu malʿūn*);[32] the Baṣran *akhbārī* al-Madāʾinī (d. 235/850) is quoted for a report about how the Umayyad caliph Sulaymān ibn ʿAbd al-Malik (r. 96–9/715–17) passed by some lepers on his way to Mecca and ordered that they be burned alive, remarking: "Had God wished that any good should come to these, He would not have tormented them with such an affliction as this."[33] Elsewhere, again free from the confining context of argument over contradictory traditions, he discusses a *ḥadīth* of the Prophet addressing the issue of whether a buyer can return to the seller a slave found to be defective in some way. Here again contagion is not explicitly mentioned, but a number of diseases from which a slave may be discovered to suffer are listed, and almost all of these are ailments considered contagious in medieval Islamic times: leprosy, consumption, and epilepsy (here called *junūn*), thus posing the dilemma of determining whether the slave already had the disease when sold to the buyer, or was infected sub-

[31] Qusṭā ibn Lūqā, *Kitāb fī l-iʿdāʾ* (Abhandlung über die Ansteckung), ed. and trans. Hartmut Fähndrich (Stuttgart: Franz Steiner Verlag, 1987).

[32] Ibn Qutayba, *ʿUyūn al-akhbār*, IV, 69:11–12.

[33] Ibid., IV, 69:13–14.

sequently.[34] It is therefore difficult to avoid the conclusion that Ibn Qutayba was a good deal closer to the pro-contagionist position, and indeed, to formal medical thinking, than his concern to defend *ḥadīth* as a discipline and source of religious knowledge would allow him openly to concede in a work in which his task was to defend *ḥadīth* from its Muʿtazilī detractors.

Our Baṣran littérateur was not alone in his ambivalent attitudes on this subject. As I have argued elsewhere, a proper understanding of medieval Islamic medicine can only be achieved by bearing in mind that the milieu in which it functioned was a profoundly pluralistic one that allowed for a wide range of medical views and practices. The formal humoral medicine had to compete with both folkloric and religious medicine, and in important ways there were overlaps and points of conjunction among the various traditions.[35] For scholars whose professional, intellectual, and personal commitments placed them astride the already ill-defined boundaries between these traditions, it was therefore difficult to adhere consistently to any one view. Al-Shāfiʿī (d. 204/819), for example, was an extremely important scholar of law whose writings on legal theory were decisive in the formulation of Islamic jurisprudence.[36] His commitments to the Qur'ān and *ḥadīth* were firm and enduring, and his career was in large part dedicated to their consecration as the ultimate sources of law and guidance for conduct by Muslims. But in a legal discussion of medical impediments to marriage his argument highlights the central role of contagious disease in such matters:

> According to what the men of medical learning and experience allege, leprosy will in many cases infect the spouse and is thus a disease dictating against sexual intercourse. Hardly any man's desire would lead him to enjoy sexual relations with a woman suffering from this disease, nor would a woman find it acceptable to have sex with a man suffering from this disease. As for the child, it is a manifest fact—but God knows best—that of

[34] Ibn Qutayba, *Al-Masā'il wa-l-ajwiba fī l-ḥadīth wa-l-tafsīr*, ed. Marwān al-ʿAṭīya and Muḥsin Kharrāba (Beirut: Dār Ibn Kathīr, 1410/1990), 35:1–4.

[35] On the interplay between these three modes of medical thought and practice in the Middle East, see Lawrence I. Conrad, "Medicine: Traditional Practice," in John L. Esposito, ed., *The Oxford Encyclopedia of the Modern Islamic World* (New York and Oxford: Oxford University Press, 1995), III, 85–9.

[36] See Christopher Melchert, *The Formation of the Sunni Schools of Law, 9th–10th Centuries* (Leiden: E. J. Brill, 1997), 68–86.

> children born to men or women who are lepers, few will be uninfected; those that do will see the disease pass on to their own children.[37]

Confronted with these facts, al-Shāfiʿī could not but concede that the infectiousness of leprosy—its "contagion"—made it impossible to allow a marriage involving a victim of this disease. Interestingly enough, he refers to medical opinion as "allegations" (*fīmā yazʿumu*), which in Islamic legal parlance means that the material being cited is open to doubt or contradicts other opinion based on better authority: i.e. he knows of the traditions being placed in circulation to deny *ʿadwā*, and is uncomfortable with the glaring contradiction between the two sides. Still, when it comes to matters of legal practice, he finds the argument for contagion too persuasive to condone a marriage between a healthy person and a leper.

Elsewhere one finds further evidence that theoretical views of contagion—i.e. arguments presented in contexts where the omnipotence of God and His will were concerned—often failed to influence actual practice. Apart from the fact that medical texts routinely upheld the doctrine of contagion,[38] public health regulations in the *ḥisba* (market inspection) treatises often presuppose the danger of the transmission of disease[39] and public authorities clearly were worried about the peril posed by lepers to healthy persons among whom they may circulate. In Cairo in 660/1262 a certificate signed by three Muslim physicians confirmed that a certain man suffered from leprosy, and so could not circulate among the Muslims "because that condition is a trans-

[37] Cited in al-Bayhaqī (d. 458/1066), *Maʿrifat al-sunan wa-l-āthār*, ed. Sayyid Kasrawī Ḥasan (Beirut: Dār al-kutub al-ʿilmīya, 1412/1991), V, 354:3–7; Ibn Ḥajar, *Badhl al-māʿūn*, 293:11–15; *idem*, *Fatḥ al-bārī*, X, 131:9–12.

[38] See, for example, al-Rāzī (d. *ca.* 313/925), *Al-Manṣūrī fī l-ṭibb*, ed. Ḥāzim al-Bakrī al-Ṣiddīqī (Kuwayt: Maʿhad al-makhṭūṭāt al-ʿarabīya, 1408/1987), 225:12–18; al-Majūsī (wr. *ca.* 363–7/973–8), *Kāmil al-ṣināʿa al-ṭibbīya* (Cairo: al-Maṭbaʿa al-kubrā al-amīrīya, AH 1294), II, 64pu–65:2; Ibn Sīnā (d. 436/1037), *Al-Qānūn fī l-ṭibb* (Cairo: al-Maṭbaʿa al-ʿāmira, AH 1294), I, 79:19–22. Cf. O. Cameron Gruner, *A Treatise on the Canon of Medicine of Avicenna* (London: Luzac, 1930), 171 no. 229.

[39] See, for example, Ibn al-Ukhūwa (d. 729/1329), *Maʿālim al-qurba fī aḥkām al-ḥisba*, ed. Muḥammad Maḥmūd Shaʿbān and Ṣiddīq Aḥmad ʿĪsā al-Muṭīʿī (Cairo: al-Hayʾa al-miṣrīya al-ʿāmma li-l-kitāb, 1976), 135:1–136ult, 154:11–12, 157:13–14, 164:4–11, 173:3–4, 178:3–4, 209:4–12, 210:3–7, 242:3.

missible and communicable disease" (*li-kawnihi mina l-amrāḍ al-mu'diya al-muntaqila*).[40]

To assert that "Islam" denies contagion is therefore to miss the essence of what was in fact a complex and difficult debate that has continued through most of Islamic history, involving contributions by individuals too numerous to consider here.[41] What stood at the heart of the matter for Muslim scholars was the problem that to accept contagion as a purely medical doctrine was to accept—at least implicitly—the possibility that things could occur in the world independent of the will of God. In some cases, it is true, scholars felt that this difficulty required the rejection of contagion in any form whatsoever. The essayist and historian Ibn al-Wardī, for example, who died in his home town of Aleppo in the late stages of the Black Death in 749/1349, survived long enough to write an essay in rhymed prose on the plague in which he categorically denied contagion and argued that God created the plague in the first place and has subsequently reconstituted it in each individual case.[42] Far more common, however, were cases in which scholars upheld the "No contagion" tradition attributed to Muḥammad, but hastened to argue that this denial applies only to claims for contagion "by its own nature", as the phrase was often put, that God often uses contagion as an instrument of His will, and that contagion in this sense is a notion that Muslims can readily accept. Both of these alternatives, as well as many others, were part of an ongoing discourse the basic problematics of which are laid out by Ibn Qutayba in clear concise form.

---

[40] See Geoffrey Khan, *Arabic Legal and Administrative Documents in the Cambridge Genizah Collections* (Cambridge: Cambridge University Press, 1993), 245–6 no. 50; discussion in H. D. Isaacs, "A Medieval Arab Medical Certificate," *Medical History* 35 (1991): 250–7.

[41] See Lawrence I. Conrad, *Contagion: the Reception of a Medical Doctrine in Islamic Society*, forthcoming.

[42] Ibn al-Wardī, *Risālat al-naba' 'an al-waba'*, reproduced in full by Ibn Ḥajar in his *Badhl al-mā'ūn*, 377pu–378:2; trans. Michael W. Dols, "Ibn al-Wardī's *Risālat al-naba' 'an al-waba'*: a Translation of a Major Source for the History of the Black Death in the Middle East," in *Near Eastern Numismatics, Iconography, Epigraphy and History: Studies in Honor of George C. Miles*, ed. Dickran K. Kouymjian (Beirut: American University of Beirut, 1974), 454.

9

Contagion and Leprosy: Myth, Ideas and Evolution in Medieval Minds and Societies

François-Olivier Touati

Leprosy and its history provide a particularly good opportunity for studying the intellectual and scientific elaboration of the notion of contagion and its implications as expressed in social behaviour, political decisions, and ways in which cultures view or represent the world. If the knowledge of the natural mode of transmission of the disease remains only a theoretical projection based on the discovery of the Hansen's bacillus (in 1873–4), and even though leprosy is today considered either non- or only slightly contagious,[1] the associations between this disease and contagion remain very strong. Indeed, in layman's parlance this disease is tantamount to contagion itself—its most highly developed metaphor, its paradigmatic exemplar.[2] This paradox illustrates the distance between reality and cultural perception, highlights the process of elaboration involved in the various ideas about contagion—the accumulated baggage of the historical heritage, and focuses our attention on three main points at least, among many other problems bearing upon the history of leprosy in the West.[3]

The first of these is the ontological connection of a specific and dated view of the Middle Ages to ideas concerning leprosy and its contagiousness. This

[1]W. A. R. Thomson, *Black's Medical Dictionary* (London: Adam and Charles Black, 1979), 525; S. R. Pattyn, P. Dockx, and J. A. Cap, *La lèpre: microbiologie, diagnostic, traitement et lutte* (Paris: Masson, 1981), 78–81; S. Kernbaum, *Eléments de pathologie infectieuse* (Paris: Specia, 1980), 438; M. D. Grmek, *Les maladies à l'aube de la civilisation occidentale* (Paris: Payot, 1983), 295–6; R. Chaussinand, *La lèpre* (Paris: Expansion scientifique française, 1955), 204; J. Maurice, "La lèpre," *La Recherche* 190 (1987): 982–91.

[2]See, for example, J.-L. Grosset and C. C. Guelpa-Lauras, "La lèpre maladie d'actualité?," in *Lèpres: Fondations Raoul Follereau* 203 (1984), 14.

[3]See the more developed analysis in my *Lèpre, lépreux et léproseries dans la province ecclésiastique de Sens jusqu'au milieu du XIVe siècle*, Doctoral thesis, Université de Paris I Panthéon–Sorbonne, 1992.

fact induced traditional historiography to remain blind—for the most part—to the possibility of elaborating a more finely nuanced perception, and instead to build up a schematic standard of interpretation or extrapolation devoid of any attention to chronology. For contemporaries, this historical discourse in turn had certain implications and effects on sanitary analyses and politics, as in the colonies, for example. Repetitions of these affirmations still validate the myth and thus impede further investigation.[4]

Second, and by extension from the above, it may be proposed that it is only through recognition of this historiographical process that we shall be able to maintain a necessary distance from traditional misinterpretations. Here, we will try to identify and to understand what can be taken to be the aetiological perceptions of leprosy as viewed through medical sources and practical usages, and the ways in which they touch upon other preoccupations in the Latin West from the fourth to the fifteenth centuries.

Third, and in order to realize these aims, special attention must be paid to chronology and to the nature of possible causes attributed to the disease, the different origins assigned to such causes, the successive and dominant choices made amongst them, and their relative characters. One must also deal with the relevant discussions that have served to promote anachronistic conclusions concerning the establishment of leper-houses and the original aims of such foundations, and recognize as such the pseudo-continuities of these institutions, falsely postulated on the basis of an apparently similar structure.

The historiographical myth

The point to be made from the outset may be summarized in fairly straightforward terms. Every consideration about leprosy and its postulated contagiousness and prevention is based on two recurrent and schematic views formulated during early modern times, reinforced during the Enlightenment, and then championed by Romantics and Positivists. The first of these makes leprosy and lepers emblematic of the dark Middle Ages. This view derives from a personalization or "heroization" of diseases into actors in history, as great scourges of humanity.[5] They are symptomatic of this demeaned period

[4]For example, J.-N. Biraben, "La maladie," in *La France médiévale*, ed. J. Favier (Paris: Fayard, 1983), 76; J. Caille, *Hôpitaux et charité publique à Narbonne au Moyen Age* (Toulouse: Société française d'histoire des hôpitaux, 1978), 33; P. Richards, *The Medieval Leper and his Northern Heirs* (Cambridge: D. S. Brewer, 1977).

[5]Illustrating this tradition is A. Cabanès, *Les fléaux de l'humanité* (Paris: A. Michel, 1920).

and are regarded as typical of a primitive civilization—an ailing and underdeveloped culture prostrated by the demise of the Roman imperium and awaiting renaissance (i.e. in the general sense of rebirth). The plague, which only demarcated the limits of the period—its beginning with the Plague of Justinian and its end with the Black Death, was insufficient for characterization of this period. Better, by far, was leprosy. Promoted by a relatively clear visibility in the sources, as compared to other undetermined diseases, leprosy perfectly symbolized these transitional times and their "degraded" status;[6] it metaphorically reflected the image of a slow rotting or swelling, a sort of chrysalis between classical Antiquity and the Renaissance,[7] and prefigured a necessary sloughing of the skin from one period to the other. It also justified—and we actually read this in Robert Moore—characterization of the medieval social order as a so-called "persecuting society".[8] This caricature lends a veneer of permanent continuity to the phenomena under investigation.

The second skewed perception is based on a polarizing equation between leprosy and contagion, lepers and rejection, and leper-houses and segregation. Each proposition infers the others, even in the absence of any evidence for one of them—specifically the first. There is clear evidence for this paradigm in most of the sources dating from the close of the Middle Ages, and modern authors, obsessed by their fear of the plague and mobilized by their rational conceptions of the new hospital and sanitary order, enforced this point of

[6]See the condemnation of medieval medicine by C. Singer, analysed by F. M. Getz in the introduction of her paper, "To Prolong Life and Promote Health: Baconian Alchemy and Pharmacy in the English Learned Tradition," in *Health, Disease and Healing in Medieval Culture*, ed. S. Campbell, B. Hall, and D. Klausner (Toronto: Macmillan, 1992), 140–1.

[7]According to C. Coury, *Histoire de la médecine* (Paris: Fayard, 1963), 324: *Tenebrae factae sunt....* See, among others, the views on this relation given by Montesquieu, *De l'esprit des lois* (Geneva: Barillot, 1748), 230; by Voltaire in his *Essai sur les mœurs* (1764), ed. J. H. Marchand (Paris: Editions sociales, 1975), 117, or in his *Questions sur l'Encyclopédie* (1774), in his *Œuvres complètes*, ed. A. J. Q. Beuchot and L. Moland, XIX (Paris: Garnier, 1879), 574, based on the *Encyclopédie*, IX (Neufchastel: S. Faulche, 1765), 395–6, the article "Léproserie" by the Chevalier de Jaucourt. On the history of the concept of the "Middle Ages" and its heavy connotation extended from the idea of the "dark" ages, see L. Gatto, *Viaggio intorno al concetto di Medioevo* (Rome: Bulzoni, 1981); J. Heers, *Le Moyen Age, une imposture* (Paris: Perrin, 1992).

[8]R. I. Moore, *The Formation of a Persecuting Society: Power and Deviance in Western Europe, 950–1250* (Oxford: Basil Blackwell, 1987), 45–65, 73–80.

view during the seventeenth and eighteenth centuries.[9] Once we have this heritage in mind, we can clearly see its resurgence in the nineteenth century: colonial politics provided an opportunity to meet other lepers, other primitives, other Middle Ages. But a special problem was posed by the resistance of native populations and cultures that espoused other attitudes or conceptions of the disease, as at Molokaï, in Indochina or among the Kanakies in New Caledonia.[10]

The reading of colonial reports concerning this resistance or contrary behaviour—sharply denounced and further fought—destroys one's absolute conviction in the monolithic perception of leprosy; it allows for the option of historicization, or more simply, it reopens historical perspectives. Contemporary observers, however, did not see this alternative, for the simple reason that it did not arise as a possibility in their minds—and indeed, was hardly a conclusion one would expect from within an imperialist context.

Unfortunately, the greater part of local erudition and scholarly publications arose in such circumstances: reflecting the current wisdom, they prejudged what the Middle Ages should have been by embracing one directed interpretation of the sources.[11] The indolent repetition of "facts" without confirming their foundation in the historical record, the usual attempts of physicians (but not historians) to write history without any basic methodology in historical research beyond a commitment to their own a priori judgements, and finally the disinclination of traditional philology to come to grips with writings in the field of medicine—all this confirmed what everyone was already convinced of. Medieval culture—conceived in terms of monolithic unity enduring for more than one thousand years, and supposedly uniform from the North Sea to the

---

[9] Excepting his introduction, strongly influenced by this historiographical tradition, which is not viewed as another form of the same discourse, see M. Foucault, *Folie et déraison: histoire de la folie à l'âge classique* (Paris: Plon, 1961).

[10] *Friend*, July 1873, 64, on which see G. Daws, *Holy Man: Father Damien of Molokaï* (New York: Harper and Row, 1973); G. Barbézieux, *Lèpre et lépreux en Indochine* (Hanoi–Haiphong: Mission d'étude, 1915); F. Ruette, *Essai sur l'éléphantiasis et les maladies lépreuses* (Paris: F. Ruette et T. Barrois, 1802), 51; P. F. O. Rayer, *Traité théorique et pratique des maladies de la peau* (Paris: J.-B. Ballière, 1826), II, 166, 306. The struggle against the natives' behaviour is described by Joseph-Siméon Roux, *Des affections lépreuses dans les régions intertropicales* (Marseille: Barlatier-Feissat, 1858), and was the subject of a documentary film on French television news (TF1, 30 January 1990).

[11] Especially with the International Congress on Leprosy since 1897. See E. Jeanselme, "Comment l'Europe au Moyen Age se protégea contre la lèpre," *Bulletin de la Société française pour l'histoire de la médecine*, 1931, 1–155; *idem*, *La lèpre* (Paris: G. Doin, 1934).

Mediterranean—was under the primary influence of the Bible and its Levitical prescriptions of "Unclean! Unclean! You will stay out of the camp!"[12] On the other hand, at the end of the period, some sources could confirm the paradigm. It was therefore sufficient to believe in the permanence of attitudes "naturally" inspired by "the" contagion, from the beginning to the end. After all, between two points only one straight line can be drawn.[13]

With respect to evidence, however, these historians did not read theology, and in particular not Jerome (345–420), Haymon of Auxerre (died c. 855), or Anselm of Laon (c. 1050–1117), who refuted the Levitical prescriptions, taking their argument from the abolition of the old Jewish law by Christ, especially concerning lepers.[14] Nor did they even take note of the comments of the great Jewish scholar Rashi himself (1040–1105) in his own highly nuanced commentaries on the same text.[15] Worse, the continuous interpolations confirmed the traditional view.

Three examples—among a long list of nonsense, anachronisms, generalizations, contradictions, or extrapolations—will serve to convey an impression of the extent of the distortions imposed on historical analysis by this recurrent paradigm.

Preserved among manuscripts written after 1200, the *Welsh Laws* by the prince Hywel Dda (d. *ca.* 950) indicates that a husband had the right to repudiate his wife if she were leprous. According to a usual reading, this passage would mean rejection and segregation of the wife, and therefore, by implica-

---

[12] Leviticus 13:45–6.

[13] For example, F. Bériac, *Histoire des lépreux au Moyen Age: une société d'exclus* (Paris: Imago, 1988), and the recent ruminations of G. Duby (about leprosy), in his "La peste, vengeance divine," in *L'Express*, 2229 (24 March 1994): 89.

[14] Jerome in his interpolated translation of Isaiah 53:44, and Gregory the Great (c. 540–604), *Homilia* XXXIX, *PL* 76, cols. 1300–1, or the emblematic representation of Job through his *Moralia, PL* 77 (especially II, 7–10, cols. 68–9); Haymon of Auxerre, *Homily of the Third Sunday after Epiphany, PL* 119, col. 138, or *Sermon for the Octave of Easter, PL* 119, cols. 493–4; Anselm of Laon, *In narrationem in Matthaeum, PL* 162, cols. 1319–20: *Cum lex prohibeat tangere leprosum, ipse solvit legem, ut Dominus se legis ostendat qui eam facit et solvere potest. Erat enim in lege permissio, non praeceptum.... Ille qui perfectionem humilitatis et misericordiae docet, destruit permissionem et docet perfectionem, ne horreamus in paupere infirmam carnem.... Quod si aliquem movet quomodo Dominus Mosaicum videtur approbare sacificium cum id non receperit Ecclesia.... Leprosus genus humanum designat....* See also the rejection by the Pope of the proposition announced by the Council of Westminster (1175–9): *Leprosi inter sanos amodo non conversentur*; M. G. Cheney, "The Council of Westminster, 1175: New Light on an Old Source," *Studies in Church History* 11 (1975): 67.

[15] See J. Bernheim, "Quarantaine pour êtres d'élite," *Tribune juive* 816 (April 1984): 30.

tion, that her affliction was regarded as contagious. But careful study of this text and comparison of its testimony with other accounts along similar lines reveals that the same attitude toward major disabilities or chronic diseases is recorded, and further, that the Church prohibited such practices. The legal conclusion in the case of the leprous wife is not her repudiation, but her protection—the restitution of her dowry (her *agweddi*).[16] The case had nothing to do with any presumed contagion.

The second example concerns the excommunications that were frequently pronounced against people who sought to be buried in the cemeteries of leprosaria. A so-called "sanitary sanction" is invoked by classical interpretation to explain this effort to intimidate possible interlopers, but how valid is this view? In reality, the only concern in such cases was to protect the rights and income of the parish from any loss, exactly as other similar religious communities sought to do when confronted by possible encroachments.[17]

A third example has to do with iconography. A famous illumination in a thirteenth-century manuscript of Vincent of Beauvais' *Miroir historial* illustrates the *Story of Barlaam and Josaphat*,[18] and shows the young Josaphat going out of his castle to meet a leper and a poor disabled man. The current title or commentary, which pays no heed to the story, or indeed, to the text on the same page, runs as follows: "A guard at the gate of a city prohibits the leper's approach."[19] In the manuscript itself, just below the illumination, the text gives exactly the opposite interpretation: Josaphat is welcoming the poor, lepers included, and the wave of his hand—a greeting of peace in the codified usage of medieval symbolism—corroborates his heart's impulse.[20] But in

[16] M. Richards, trans., *The Laws of Hywel Dda (The Book of Blegywryd)* (Liverpool: University of Liverpool Press, 1954), 69 (also 46, 99, to compare the lepers' status with that of other sick or religious people); full texts with references to the Welsh legislation and canonical dispositions in J. Y. Simpson, "On Leprosy and Leper Hospitals in Scotland and England," in his *Archaeological Essays*, ed. J. Stuart, with additional notes by J. Robertson (Edinburgh: Edmonston and Douglas, 1872), 173–6.

[17] For example, at Melun in 1160: Arch. dep. Seine-et-Marne H 222, ed. and commentaries by G. Leroy in *Revue des sociétés savantes* 3 (1866): 301–2; also at Aberdeen: Robertson, "Additional Notes," 172; and after the decisions of the Council of Latran III (1179), the recall by the Council of Westminster (1200): J. D. Mansi, ed., *Sacrorum conciliorum nova et amplissima collectio* (Florence: A. Zatta, 1759–98), XXII, cols. 719–20, cap. xiii.

[18] Bibliothèque nationale (Paris), Ms. Arsenal 5080 Rés., fol. 373r.

[19] Jeanselme, *La lèpre*, 48; or more recently, R. Delort, *Le Moyen Age: histoire illustrée de la vie quotidienne* (Paris: Le Seuil, 1972), 52.

[20] *L'Histoire de Barlaam et Josaphat* (version champenoise), ed. L. R. Mills (Geneva: Droz, 1973), 46–8.

such circumstances, why does the leper have his traditional clapper, if not to warn away the healthy? Before changing its significance and use, succeeding to the horn (the "flavel"), the clapper or the bell (on the *Exeter Pontifical*, for instance, where a marginal sketch showing a leper with a bell is joined with the following phylactery from his mouth: "[s-]um good my gentyll mayster for God sake") represented an effort to compensate for the leper's voice deficiency: all twelfth and thirteenth-century accounts of lepers in chronicles and other texts, and some of those from the fourteenth century, attest to the clapper's function of calling people's attention to the proximity of someone who needed to beg from them—the aim was to attract them, not to drive them away.[21]

These simple examples must cause us to doubt old traditional ideas, however venerable; they oblige us to look at the problem afresh from a different viewpoint and to renounce questionable evidence. In these circumstances, how should we consider the aetiological perception of leprosy over the long term and through the diversity of countries that comprised medieval Europe? Contagion? What contagion?

Leprosy, contagion and medical writings

In order to understand the possible causes assigned to leprosy by medieval physicians, it is first necessary to bear in mind the conception of the disease itself.

From Celsus or Galen—speaking about elephantiasis—to Henry of Mondeville at least, in the fourteenth century, leprosy was categorized as a chronic affliction: "heavy and serious" for Rufus of Ephesus in the second century or Oribasius in the fourth, "incurable and violent" for Lanfrancus (before 1296) or Henry of Mondeville (in 1304–6).[22] Far from being classified among the cutaneous diseases, as was the case in nineteenth-century

[21] British Library (London), Ms. Lansdowne 451, fol. 123r, reproduced in Richards, *The Medieval Leper*, 52; Guillaume of Saint-Pathus, *Vie de Saint Louis*, ed. H.-F. Delaborde (Paris: Imprimerie nationale, 1899), 107–8; other references in Touati, *Lèpre, lépreux et léproseries*, 711–15.

[22] Celsus, *De medicina* III.25; Galen, *Ad Glauconem de medendi methodo* II, XII; Oribasius, *Collectio medica* XLV.28; Lanfrancus, *Practica* (Venice: Juntas, 1546), fol. 227v (= *En cyrurgie*, ed. G. Yvoire, Lyon: J. de la Fontaine, 1490, III.7); Mondeville, *Chirurgia*, ed. J. L. Pagel, *Die Chirurgie des Heinrich von Mondeville* (Berlin: G. Reimer, 1892), x–xi, 423. See our more detailed discussion in *Lèpre, lépreux et léproseries*, 362–84; also J. G. Andersen, "Studies in the Mediaeval Diagnosis of Leprosy in Denmark," *Danish Medical Bulletin* 16 (1969), Suppl. IX.

academic discourse and nosology, leprosy was only compared to them, as well as other partially and symptomatically similar afflictions (pneumonic flow for respiratory lesions, for instance), precisely for a differential diagnostic from diseases with similar symptoms. With Isidore of Seville in the seventh century, Rabanus Maurus in the ninth, or in the manuscripts of Chartres in the tenth, we find such phrases as "leprosy of the flesh and the skin" and "leprosy of the entire body", a pathology described from an internal part, from viscera extended to the superficial parts.[23] Described as an attack on the whole structure of the body, all members and organs included, leprosy had the same nature as cancer, according to Constantine the African, following Galen.[24] Based on Theodoricus (1205–98), Mondeville provides its most comprehensive definition:

> Leprosy is a hideous disease... originated from melancholy or matter transformed in melancholy, corrupted by an irradicable corruption (*corruptione incorrigibili*), and it is to the entire body what a cancer is to the cancerous member (*quasi cancer membro cancerato*)....[25]

This view, implicitly or explicitly dependent on Galen's humoral system, leads us to the essential explanation of the disease: the integrity of the flesh, originating in blood, and the composition of the body, originating in humours (or more specifically, generated from their secondary products—sperm and menstrual blood), can be placed in danger should there occur a disruption of its metamorphosis, leading to a plethora of blood and an ensuing imbalance of the different humours. If for one reason or another there should occur a "great error in the property of assimilation", as explained by Constantine or Lanfrancus—which is to say, bad digestion in a wide sense, or if there should be bad circulation of the humours, bad evacuation (in menstruation, for instance), bad excretion imputed to a bad dietetic regime (gluttony, according

[23] *PL* 83, col. 328: ... *in carne et cute gerunt lepram, qui carnalia vel exteriora suadere conantur....*; *De universo, PL* 111, col. 502: *Leprosi toto in corpore....*; Bibliothèque municipale de Chartres, Ms. 62, fol. 102r—cf. L. C. MacKinney, "Tenth-Century Medicine as Seen in the *Historia* of Richer of Rheims," *Bulletin of the History of Medicine* 2 (1934): 369 n. 56.

[24] *Ad Glauconem*, II, XII; *Pantegni*, ed. in *Omnia opera Ysaac... cum quibusdam aliis opusculis* (Lyon: Bartholomeus Trot, 1515), *Theorica* VIII.15, fol. 39v; *Viaticum* VII.17.

[25] *Chirurgia*, 422; Theodoricus, *Chirurgia* (Venice: Juntas, 1546), fol. 178r: *Fit autem lepra de materia melancholica inculcata in tota carne et in cute exterius....*; Lanfrancus, *Practica*, fol. 227v: *Et est toti corpori sicut cancer existit in uno membro....*

to Hildegard of Bingen in the twelfth century), or absence of fasting or purging, then an "accumulation of bad blood" (Giles of Corbeil) will result.[26] If such an accumulation is not evacuated quickly with the help of medicine or nature (as in menstruation), it will generate "monstrous pains", according to Bartholomaeus Anglicus (d. *ca.* 1240–50).[27] Aggravated by abuses over the course of time, this superfluity can never be palliated by the regulative organs, such as the liver, the spleen, or even the pores of the skin. According to Mondeville, a "putrefaction" or "combustion" will eventually cause the accumulation to transform itself into a melancholic humour "contrary to nature and life".[28] Instead of remaining localized, as in the case of haemorrhoids, or at the breast, as in cancer, this melancholy taints or corrupts the blood and, by "sympathy", impregnates the whole flesh, the skin and the other humours, obstructing the process of humoral excretion. In all four of the main types into which leprosy was classified (*elephantia*, *leonina*, *thiria*, and *alopecia*), depending on which of the four humours was believed to have been at fault, the melancholy comes to dominate the whole humoral system with a venomous poison[29] that eventually extends to its spermatic product. In this way, and especially in the case of a disease that requires some time before revealing symptoms, it becomes easy to understand how the idea of contagion—in its modern sense of pathogenic transmission—might remain secondary for a long time. Indeed, not in any case has it ever been regarded as the exclusive cause of leprosy.

Though certain historians or naturalists wrote otherwise, the ancient medical authorities who comprised the founts of knowledge during the Middle Ages—Celsus, Rufus, and Oribasius, for example—refute the idea of propagation of the disease. And for Galen, if the "initial cause is external to the body, it will not have any effect without a previous cause, that is to say, without bodily predisposition".[30] Only Areteus the Cappadocian in the

---

[26] Constantine the African, *Pantegni*, *Theorica* VIII.15, fol. 39v: . . . *Quae concreatur cumque in carne est deficiat mutativa virtus*; Lanfrancus, *Chirurgia*, fol. 227v; Hildegard of Bingen, *Causae et curae*, ed. P. Kaiser (Leipzig: Teubner, 1903), 18, 160; Giles of Corbeil, *Viaticus*, ed. V. Rose (Leipzig: Teubner, 1906), 74: . . . *lepra pluribus ex causis oritur, generante diaeta sanguinis inmundi cumulum*. . . .

[27] *De proprietatibus rerum* (Basle: M. Wenssler, 1475), fol. 19r.

[28] *Chirurgia*, 429–30.

[29] For example, *Glosule quattuor magistrorum*, ed. S. De Renzi in *Collectio salernitana* (Naples: Filiatre-Sebezio, 1853), II, 703–4.

[30] M. D. Grmek, "Le concept d'infection dans l'Antiquité et au Moyen Age: les anciennes mesures sociales contre les maladies contagieuses et la fondation de la première quarantaine à

first century—without any influence on the West—and Caelius Aurelianus, between the third and the fifth centuries, discussed a "fear of living" with lepers, or fear of "colouring" (*infectio* in Latin, *baphē* in Greek) by breathing.[31] And when, especially from the thirteenth century onward, authors like Lanfrancus remarked "how the breath and perspiration of lepers stink", they were in the first instance emphasizing a particular symptom, not a supposed cause.[32] One must bear in mind at all times that the chronological priority of a certain viewpoint does not suggest, much less prove, anything as to its further reception in later times, and that the same word may be used by different authors in different senses.

The vocabulary used in most medical writings indicates that the horrifying visual aspect of leprosy impressed the most experienced practitioners; but even so, one does not find this translating into some hypothetic fear of contamination. The term "contagion" is only and simply a synonym for the notion of "disease", according to Gregory of Tours, who employed it in the sixth century independently from any mention of leprosy. It may also be noted here that all of his descriptions of lepers situate these poor meeting the saint or going to the sanctuaries along with other people.[33] The notion of "contagion", still used by Giles of Corbeil at the end of the twelfth century, belongs to the same category as "infection", "corruption", or "putrefaction"; it is applied to the internal and pathological process in which the body slowly becomes impregnated with venomous humour, leading to the destruction of the whole edifice (*templum naturae perimens contagio lepra. . . .*). It refers essentially to the

Dubrovnik (1377)," *Rad. Jugoslavenska Akademija znanosti i umjetnosti* (Zagreb) 384 (1980): 9–54; *idem*, "Les vicissitudes des notions d'infection, de contagion et de germe dans la médecine antique," *Mémoires du Centre J. Palerne (Saint-Etienne)* 3 (1984): 53–70; J.-M. André, "L'épidémiologie de Pline," in *Pline l'Ancien, témoin de son temps*, ed. J. Pigeaud and J. Oroz Reta (Salamanca and Nantes: Universidad Pontificia de Salamanca, 1987), 42–52; V. Nutton, "The Seeds of Disease: an Explanation of Contagion and Infection from the Greeks to the Renaissance," *Medical History* 27 (1983): 1–34, esp. 15: "the seeds of disease... would play only a minor role at best".

[31] Grmek, "Le concept d'infection," 15–16; H. E. Sigerist, "Early Mediaeval Medical Texts in Manuscripts of Vendôme," *Bulletin of the History of Medicine* 14 (1943): 68–89. See the expression of the *Roman de Rou*, written by Wace *ca.* 1160, ed. A. J. Holden (Paris: Société des anciens textes français, 1970), II, 239: "Rou estoit de liepre tuz teinz et tuz vertiz."

[32] Lanfrancus, *Chirurgia*, fol. 227v: *Item anhelitus eis foeret, et sudor.* See also the Old French version of 1490, *En cyrurgie* III.i.7; and the Old English version, *Chirurgie*, ed. R. v. Fleischhacker (London: K. Paul, Trench, Trübner and Co., 1894), 197.

[33] *De virtutibus S. Martini* IV.46: *Advenerat quidam ex Brittania qui caecus, mutus ac surdus, manibus contractus per quoddam contagio fuerat.*

progression of leprosy, originated in the body itself,[34] while the recognition of transmissibility from one person to another supposes an abstract separation between the disease and the body or individual who carries it. A number of difficulties militated against this dichotomy: the epidemiology of leprosy, the absence of any conceptual or material input from bacteriology, and the propensity of humoral theory for consideration of the body and human pathology as a closed universe. The whole question highlights the issue of the forms of exchange between scientific writings and works of other kinds; it puts forward the problem of the constitution, transmission, and reception of medical discourses, along with all their falterings, debates, and contradictions.

Arguments on the possible causes of leprosy were more problematic, as they turned precisely on those realities that were still difficult to observe empirically. "We can still identify leprosy only a long time after its invasion of the body," said Constantine the African at the end of the eleventh century; he goes on to recognize that "from this point, the search for its origin is difficult and arduous".[35] One may well admire him for his astute observation on how the onset of the disease long precedes the appearance of its symptoms, but here the word "invasion", like the term "contagion", must not be allowed to deceive us. It concerns the process of clinical development from an original phase, not an aetiology or cause explained at distance.[36] The interpretation of these causes thus remains especially dependent upon cultural circumstances; it is influenced by the interplay of other discourses and subject to the ambiguous superimposition of different paradigms and possible variants.

Could the example of the plague or various other pestilences, and in particular Galen's explanation of the causes of the famous Athenian Plague—a *locus classicus* for Greek and Latin authors—provide a schema, even if only implicitly, for the aetiological perception of leprosy? Galen's commentary in-

[34] Giles of Corbeil, *Viaticus*, 74; Mondeville, *Chirurgia*, 429–30: ... *in causa imediata cujus libet speciei leprae est solus humor melancholicus venenosus horribilis et infectus, quod natura non potest ipsum assimilare cum carne bona et ideo fit lepra... et est hujusmodi melancholia putrefacta non putrefactione faciente saniem sicut in apostematibus nec putrefactione fluidorum liquidorum, quae faciunt febrem, sed putrefactione que est adustio et incineratio.*

[35] Constantine the African, *Pantegni, Practica* IV.2, fol. 93r; *idem, Liber aureus* (Basle: H. Petrus, 1536), 187 (Cap. XLVII): *Lepra difficilis est ad curandum et hoc ideo quia cum cognoscitur diu est quod corpus invasit. In initio enim et nimis post initium non potest cognosci.*

[36] On this vocabulary, see D. Gourévitch, "Les faux-amis dans les textes médicaux grecs et latins," in *Mémoires du Centre J. Palerne (Saint-Etienne)* 3 (1982): 189–91; *idem*, "Peut-on employer le mot d'infection dans les traductions françaises des textes latins?," *Mémoires du Centre J. Palerne (Saint-Etienne)* 5 (1984): 49–52.

troduced the notion of seeds in corrupted air. To be accepted, the hypothesis of this aetiological analogy with leprosy would imply that leprosy occurs like a ravaging pandemic. But no physician was prepared to lend credence to this comparison. In the seventh century, Isidore of Seville gave a complete definition of pestilence: "When caught by one, it has already passed on the others because it comes from impure air and penetrates the body."[37] Yet a whole chapter on chronic diseases separates this sentence from the discussion of leprosy. Still in the thirteenth century or at the beginning of the fourteenth, physicians such as John of Saint-Amand or Maynus of Mayneris, speaking about epidemics, invoked the notion of pestilential air without drawing a connection with leprosy.[38]

Even if the aetiological comparison with plague is accepted, however, one would still be obliged to address the problem of how practitioners dealt with the highly disconcerting question (also evident in Galen's approach to epidemic disease) of why "all people exposed to this air do not fall ill"?[39] Based on Theodoricus, Lanfrancus in the thirteenth century commented on leprosy in these terms: "It passes from one to another and from father to son, but not always, because sometimes a healthy person who lives with a leper does not become leprous, and a leper can give birth to someone who will not be leprous. . . ."[40] The relative aspect of contagiousness could hardly find clearer expression. At the beginning of the thirteenth century, Gilbert the Englishman has this information to offer in his famous *Compendium medicinae*: "Physicians are discussing material causes of leprosy, but not characteristics of leprosy."[41]

By deploying a double aetiology in which the initial pollution by an external agent acts in accordance with an individual's own prior predisposition,

---

[37] *De medicina* IV.6–8, *PL* 176, col. 187.

[38] John of Saint-Amand, *Concordanciae*, ed. J. L. Pagel (Berlin: G. Reimer, 1894), 93, 116; Maynus of Mayneris [Magninus Mediolanensis], *Regimen sanitatis* (Lyon: J. Myt., 1517), fol. 92r, on *Signa pestilentia.*

[39] Grmek, "Vicissitudes," 62.

[40] *Chirurgia* III.7: . . . *transit de uno ad alium et hereditatur, licet haec duo semper non sint necessaria nam aliquando sanus conversatur cum leproso, nec inficitur, et leprosus poteste etiam sanum generare. . . .* The Old French version is clearer: ". . . elle va de l'ung a l'autre et de hoir en hoir iassoit ce que non pas tousiours car aucune fois [quelquefois] personne qui est saine converse avec ung lépreux et par ce n'est pas faict lepreix at aussi ung lépreux peut bien engendrer ung qui ne sera pas lépreux. . . ." See also Theodoricus, *Chirurgia*, fol. 178r.

[41] Gilbert the Englishman, *Compendium medicinae* (Lyon: J. Saccon, 1510), fol. 337r: *Medici autem disputant de causis materialibus lepre et non de egritudine que est lepra.*

the physicians' explanation followed the Galenic paradigm. There could be putrefaction, "colouring", or impregnation—medieval terms for the notion of pathological evolution—only if residual matter carried by humours arose from a "stoppage of ducts", a default of perspiration (elimination), a "plethora", or an "excess of food, drink and sexual intercourse, with inevitable digestive disorders".[42] This system could encompass the miasmatic aetiology, but turned it on its head and, as articulated by John of Saint-Amand and others, argued for the body's capacity to assimilate and eliminate external or corrupted matter. All depended on the condition of the body: the disease could simply have its origin in dysfunction that leads to engorgement and the prevalence of one humour—mainly melancholy—and to dyscrasia. To maintain good health, one had not to beware of contaminating contact with lepers, but to protect oneself from possible abuses. Among such abuses, a quite frequently invoked culprit was food absorbed in excess or eventually corrupted, especially food analogically related to each humour, following the form of leprosy, melancholy, or phlegmatic temperament, for example.[43] In the same way, immoderate sexual behaviour was considered capable of producing a dangerous superfluity by venereal accumulation or conception with hereditarily corrupted sperm (according to Constantine, Theodoricus, or Albertus Magnus).[44] In theory, the humoral denominator of these causes explains perfectly this indissociable relation between the congenital, the venereal, and ideas about "contagion" in the sense of impregnation from one humour to another.[45] William of Conches, at the beginning of the eleventh century, had

[42]Cf. Galen, *De febrium differentiis* I.6, ed. C. G. Kühn (Leipzig: Teubner, 1821–33), VII, 289–91.

[43]For instance, Giles of Corbeil, *Viaticus*, 74–5, v. 1831–6; Aldebrandinus of Siena (living at Troyes, Champagne, in the second half of the thirteenth c.), *Le régime du corps*, ed. L. Landouzy and R. Pépin (Paris: H. Champion, 1911), 123, 129.

[44]Constantine the African, *Pantegni*: *Theorica* VIII.15: *Est autem de complexione mala, frigida et sicca et de dominatione melancholie ad sanguinem et corruptione eiusdem.... Substantia enim spermatis commixta est cum humoribus malis de quibus lepra procretur....*; *Chirurgia* III.15, fol. 178v: *... sicut ex parentela et est morbus hereditarius. Item generatur in matrice, menstruis immundis repleta, licet semina sint munda....*; Albertus Magnus, *Quaestiones super de animalibus* XV.13, ed. E. Filthaut as *Alberti Magni Opera omnia*, XII (Münster: Aschendorf, 1951), 267: *... unde sperma leprosi est infectum, et ideo consimilis est infectio in foetu.*

[45]Constantine the African, *Pantegni*: *Theorica* VIII.15: *... Que cum veniat ad corporis nutrimenta corrumpit ea et dessicat et ita corrumpit humores corporis atque sperma....* See the stimulating study by S. R. Ell, "Blood and Sexuality in Medieval Leprosy," *Janus* 71 (1984): 153–64, and with reservations about the confusion of leprosy with other diseases (Nicolas–Favre syndrome), D. Jacquart and C. Thomasset, *Sexualité et savoir médical au Moyen Age* (Paris: Presses

no other explanation in the case of podagra, for example.[46] But more practically, only the long duration of these abuses, with their repetition inducing a slow impregnation, seemed to favour the disease: Giles of Corbeil insisted on this determining factor.[47] And only a long relationship with lepers—in family circles, in communal relations, or in sexuality—was able to provoke the disease. Practitioners probably had occasion to observe the coincidence in cases within a family, but they would have seen the opposite as well! This is why, when confronted with the possibility of such a spread of leprosy, medical writings were reserved, articulating preferentially and without any sense of hierarchy the different elements considered to influence the appearance of the disease. Considering this wide choice of options, direct and personal contamination by simple contact, not to mention transmission through the air, failed to gain wide acceptance for the simple reason that pre-existing theoretical structures allowed it only marginal credibility.

However, in the decade from 1220 to 1230 there are some indications of a progressive changing perception. These echo the advanced discussions not of physicians, but of other authorities, the experts in canon law, and most especially deal with a question of marriage law—the right of lepers to live or not to live with their legal wife or husband. In his *Summa aurea*, Henry of Suse wrote in 1253: "Some distinguish a contagious leprosy, but not unanimously, from another that is not contagious."[48] Here the verb *inficere*, which we have translated as "contagious", has certainly acquired the new sense that we have come to anticipate in modern times.

Leaving aside the question of social factors, one must recognize the new and important influence of Arab-Islamic medicine on the Latin West. If at first discreet, later, after the appearance of most of the leper-houses, its contribution to the debate about leprosy was to become very important indeed.

universitaires de France, 1985), 242–64; analysis in our review of the book, *Revue de Synthèse*, Quatrième Série, 3 (1986): 325–6, and our article "Facies leprosorum: réflexions sur le diagnostic facial de la lèpre au Moyen Age," *Histoire des sciences médicales* 20 (1986): 57–66; also L. Demaitre, "The Description and Diagnosis of Leprosy by Fourteenth-Century Physicians," *Bulletin of the History of Medicine* 59 (1985): 331–4.

[46] William of Conches, *De philosophia mundi*, *PL* 90, col. 1170 (Pseudo-Bede); see B. Lawn, *The Salernitan Questions* (Oxford: Clarendon Press, 1963), 53–4 (notes).

[47] *Viaticus*, 75 v. 1840–1.

[48] Henry of Suse, *Summa aurea* (Basle: T. Guarinum, 1573), IV, col. 1048: *Alii distingunt inter lepram quae inficit, ut tunc cogatur praecise... et lepram quae non inficit....* On this important author, who was archdeacon of Paris and teacher before the highest dignities, see N. Didier, "Henri de Suse, prieur d'Antibes," in *Studia Gratiana* 2 (1954) 608–17.

Even if the Middle Eastern physicians were not unanimous about the transmission of diseases, and especially leprosy,[49] some Arabic texts translated into Latin for the first time by Constantine the African in Italy and Gerard of Cremona in Spain were able to explain the subject more clearly.[50] In the *Theorica* section of the *Pantegni* (translated from the *Kāmil al-ṣināʿa al-ṭibbīya* of al-Majūsī), Constantine described the humoral origin of leprosy, argued for its hereditary transmission, and then stated: "In the same, some people are touched [by leprosy] from living and speaking with lepers. Indeed, noxious fumes coming from the dissolution of sick bodies are inhaled by healthy people."[51] And further in the *Practica* one reads: "The cause of this putrefaction comes from corrupted sperm, male or female or both, or from corruption of the air or food and drink. . . ."[52]

This new factor of corruption of the air is here linked to leprosy for the first time. But the immediate impact of this formulation is far from certain, even with the obvious concession that Constantine's translation played a decisive part in the constitution of Western medicine. The passage is but a brief statement in a vast work, and its juxtaposition in context with other possible factors did not favour its easy assimilation into the humoral interpretation of leprosy; it was often absent from Latin manuscripts,[53] and the *Pantegni* itself, criticized for other reasons, fell into discredit and was excluded from university programmes. By comparison, Constantine's other more successful works—the *Ysagoge*, the *De melancholia*, and the *Viaticum*, all of which were widely circulated and used in teaching—are absolutely silent on the contagiousness of leprosy.[54]

---

[49] See in this book the analysis by L. I. Conrad; also M. W. Dols, "Leprosy in Medieval Arabic Medicine," *Journal of the History of Medicine* 34 (1979): 314–33 (conclusion, 331); *idem*, "The Leper in Medieval Islamic Society," *Speculum* 58 (1983): 891–916.

[50] On the transmission to the Latin West, see D. Jacquart and F. Micheau, *La médecine arabe et l'occident médiéval* (Paris: Maisonneuve et Larose, 1990).

[51] *Pantegni*: *Theorica* VIII.15: . . . *Item occupantur quidam cum sani huiusmodi assideant et eis confabulentur. Malus enim fumus de corporibus infirmis dissolutus a sanis odoratur*. . . .

[52] *Pantegni*: *Practica* IV.2, fol. 93r: . . . *Putredinum autem causa aut ex corruptione et spermatis masculis sive utriusque aut ex corruptione aeris sive cibi et potus*. . . .

[53] For example, Bibliothèque Nationale (Paris), Ms. Latin 13,000 (from Saint-Germain-des-Prés).

[54] Constantine the African, *Ysagoge*, in his *Opera* (Basle: H. Petrus, 1536), 187, from Ḥunayn ibn Isḥāq—see G. Maurach, ed., "Johannicius, Isagoge ad Techne Galieni," *Sudhoffs Archiv* 62 (1978): 148–74; *idem*, *De melancholia libri duo*, ed. K. Garbers (Hamburg: Buske, 1977), 192–3; *idem*, *Viaticum* (Lyon: Bartholomeus Trot, 1515), fol. 170r.

Avicenna's *Canon*, translated at Toledo before 1187, provides a more developed account. In the part of Book IV devoted to leprosy, one chapter describes the humoral characteristics of the disease and attributes its origin primarily to an increasing flow of black bile impregnating each "member" (i.e. the organs) via blood and phlegm. Two kinds of causes explain this disorder. First, there is the antecedent cause, a faulty complexion of the liver; in that case, phlegmatic and plethoric food is incriminated. The second cause is a consequence of the first: the inability of the spleen to purify the blood, or the vitiation of the capacities of elimination, debilitating the viscera, sphincters, womb, and pores. Lastly, a third type of cause, considered as adjuvant only, is invoked:

> And sometimes, says Avicenna, the air, corrupted in itself or by reason of the proximity of lepers, adds to all this because the disease is contagious. And sometimes the disease arises by heredity, or by the embryo's complexion being defectively formed and given, or is acquired by the disposition of the womb in the case of menstrual conception; sometimes leprosy comes from hot air joined to bad food—salted fish and meat, coarse meat, and donkey meat, lentils certainly—as it develops in Alexandria. . . .[55]

Leprosy is cited again in Book I of the *Canon*, in a list of certain diseases that "pass from one to another": it is associated with scabies, smallpox, pestilential fevers, and purulent ulcers, and in the cases of ophthalmia and phthisis it is linked to the direction of the wind and the insalubrity of houses. Following this first list, leprosy is also mentioned among the hereditary diseases, after white herpes or eczema, baldness, podagra and phthisis.[56]

Apart from the fact that these passages are brief, relatively isolated and without consequence in any hypothetical segregation of those affected by these other diseases, it is to be noted that Avicenna's purposes are finely nuanced.

[55] *Liber Canonis* (Venice: L. A. Giunta, 1527), IV.iii.3, fol. 346r.b: . . . *Et quandoque adiuvat illud totum corruptio aeris in se ipso, aut propter vicinitatem leprosorum, quoniam aegritudo est* [*contagiosa*] *invadens. Et quandoque accidit propter haereditatem, et propter complexionem* [*alnathe*] *embryonis ex qua erratus est in seipso propter complexionem, qua est ei, aut acquisitam in matrice, propter dispositionem quae est ei: sicut si accipiat ei ut sit conceptio in dispositione menstruorum, et quando aggregatur calidas aeris cum malitia cibi, et eius essentia ex genere piscium et carne salita, et carne grossa, et carnibus asinorum, et lentibus proculdubio est ut eveniat lepra: sicut multiplicatur in Alexandria. . . .*

[56] *Liber Canonis*, I.ii.1, 8, fols. 23v.b, 24r.a.

His text deliberately and comprehensively follows a hierarchical order: the dyscrasia is linked to the predispositions of the body and with the internal increase of the disease, before there is any enumeration of other possible factors having to do with the environment or eventual contamination. The idea of accumulation confirms the humoral explanation, and one must note that Avicenna does not warn against the eventual corruption of food with which lepers have come into contact—indeed, within a humoral context this would perhaps have been difficult to visualize and accept.

Now, would this more explicit message have had the effect of promoting the notion of an aerial aetiology and hence a perception of the peril of coming into contact with lepers? Even though the thesis was now more clearly articulated, the answer to this question would seem to have been no, at least at first. The position of this cause, among a wide choice of others, led medical authorities only to recognize it as adjuvant: Lanfrancus repeated it word for word, considering all its relative aspects, and not many physicians or others used this argument before the end of the thirteenth century. The reception of the *Canon* was slow, and its first attested reader in northern Europe was Girard of Bourges, who in his *Commentary* on the *Viaticus* of Constantine, written between 1230 and 1237, spoke in his chapter on leprosy only about the hereditary and sexual transmission of the disease, following the humoral schema.[57] At the most, in circumstances that had become unfavourable to lepers, this focusing of aetiology provided an opportunity for an elaborate discussion between moralists and physicians, at a time of new debates opened by Aristotelianism and Averroism precisely on the issue of corruption and generation.[58] Only a single manuscript, belonging to the Chapter of Notre-Dame of Paris at the time of Girard of Bourges, invokes the argument of aerial contamination in seeking to demonstrate the contagiousness of a leper's

[57] Girard of Bourges, *Glosule super Viaticum Constantini*, Bibliothèque Nationale (Paris), Ms. Latin 6888, fols. 99v–100r, and Ms. Latin 6889, fol. 186v; D. Jacquart, "La réception du *Canon* d'Avicenne: comparaison entre Montpellier et Paris aux XIIIe et XIVe siècles," *Histoire de l'école médicale de Montpellier: Actes du 110e Congrès national des sociétés savantes* (Paris: Comité des travaux historiques et scientifiques, 1985), 69–77.

[58] Averroes, *Commentarium medium in Aristotelis De generatione et corruptione libros*, ed. F. H. Fobes (Cambridge, Mass.: Medieval Academy of America, 1956). On the polemics, which mainly concerned Paris and Oxford, see R. Hissette, *Enquête sur les 219 articles condamnés à Paris le 7 mars 1277* (Louvain and Paris: Vander-Oyez, 1977); F. van Steenberghen, *Aristote en Occident* (Louvain: Institut Supérieur de Philosophie, 1946); A. Hewson, *Giles of Rome and the Theory of Conception* (London: Athlone Press, 1975).

glance at a child.[59] This unique example, probably arising from an over-hasty reading of the *Canon* and from an insufficient assimilation of its connection between leprosy and ophthalmia, demonstrates the misapprehension of the aerial aetiology.

About ten years later, the book devoted to medicine in an encyclopedic work by a Franciscan who was probably not a physician, but a theologian, Bartholomaeus Anglicus, illustrates the balance between the traditional conceptions of leprosy and the new acceptance of its contagiousness.[60] In his text, Bartholomaeus first draws a clearer distinction between the humoral nature or growth of the disease (explicitly following Constantine) and its "various causes", which are themselves classified into two categories. Some causes are sexual or hereditary: the disease can arise from the bad blood of a parent, or can come about during menstruation or the feeding of the child by a leprous mother.[61] Other causes are extrinsic: the disease can arise by way of putrid air, bad food (on which some new details are given: abuse of garlic or pepper, pork infected with "granules", corrupted wine), or even the bite of reptiles. The list is still presented as an enumeration of eventualities "besides the aforementioned humours", without any precision about the origin of the air. But, as put forward and covering all these factors, it begins with the consideration of living, eating and frequent association with lepers, "because the disease is contagious and infects others".[62] This pleonasm reflected the recent acceptance of a less traditional sense for the notion of contagion, and called for a pedagogical definition: "contagious, that is to say, infective from one to another", Bartholomaeus seems obliged to insist. But if the notion had really been assimilated, would it have been necessary or useful to repeat it and explain the signification of the word?

[59] *The Prose Salernitan Questions*, ed. B. Lawn (Oxford: Oxford University Press, 1979), 98, B, q. 179.

[60] *De proprietatibus rerum*, fols. 66v.a–67r.b.

[61] *Ibid.*, fol. 67r.a: . . . *Aliquando etiam accidit quando concipitur fetus tempore menstruorum vel quando ex corrupto lacte mulieris leprose nutritur fetus*. . . . According to the humoral system, the "milk" was deemed a product of humours and qualifies here the alimentation during gestation; it has nothing to do with the erroneous translation given by S. Rubin, *Medieval English Medicine* (London and New York: Barnes and Noble, 1974), 153: "feeding a child with the milk of a leprous nurse".

[62] *Ibid.*, fol. 67r.a: . . . *Nascitur autem lepra a causis variis preterquam ab humoribus predictis, sicut ex cohabitacione et convictu et frequenti confabulatione cum leprosis: contagiosus enim est morbus et aliorum infectivus*. . . .

On the whole, however, physicians were not ready to privilege this factor, and the new texts that came to be known during the second half of the thirteenth century—such as Rhazes' or Avicenna's *Cantica*—were not more favourable to this opinion.[63] The success itself of Bartholomaeus' *De proprietate rerum* ("On the Properties of Things") would come later, with translations into French and English.[64] Still, the growth of Avicenna's authority at the end of the thirteenth century, already before its consecration in the fourteenth, makes this point more and more difficult to avoid, whatever its detractors or the distance between the theory and the reality: an "arduous subject", Mondeville recognized at the beginning of the fourteenth century.[65]

It was only at this time, in conjunction with other social, economic, and religious considerations, that medical writings began to mark a progressive evolution. With Bernard of Gordon and John of Gaddesden, for example, Pietro of Abano in his famous *Conciliator* points in original terms to "corrupted and pestilential air" as ranking among predispositions to leprosy; however, he does not specify whether the origin of this "air" is natural or human.[66] Another contemporary text, the *Breviarium practicae*, probably Italian but long erroneously ascribed to Arnaldus of Villanova, provides further details on air contamination. For the first time in medical writing, to my knowledge, it draws inferences by way of explaining the henceforth imposed segregation of lepers.[67] Still, this firm position contradicts the more common reticence

[63] Avicenna, *Poème de la médecine*, ed. and trans. H. Jahier and A. Noureddine (Paris: Société d'édition "Les Belles Lettres", 1956), 179; Rhazes, *Liber ad Almansorem* (Basle: H. Petrus, 1544), 96, 422–3; *idem, Antidotis liber* (Basle: H. Petrus, 1544), 455; *idem, Guide du médecin nomade: aphorisms*, trans. E. Moubachir (Paris: Sindbad, 1980), 61, 83, 98. See Dols, "Leprosy in Medieval Arabic Medicine," 331.

[64] C. Herfray-Rey, "Jean Corbechon, traducteur de Barthélemy l'Anglais (1372)," in *Ecole nationale des Chartes: Position des thèses* (Paris: Ecole nationale des Chartes, 1944), 59–61; *On the Properties of Things: John Trevisa's Translation of Bartholomaeus Anglicus' "De proprietate rerum"*, ed. M. C. Seymour *et al.* (Oxford: Clarendon Press, 1975–88).

[65] *Chirurgia*, 428.

[66] Pietro of Abano, *Conciliator* (Mantua, 1472), Diff. 177: *... aut ab aere corrupto pestilentiali... vel propter moram cum leprosis....*; Bernard of Gordon, *Lilium medicinae* (Lyon: G. Rouillius, 1550), 89, seeming, nevertheless, to have a doubt: *... hoc potest esse quia aer est malus corruptus, pestilentialis....*; John of Gaddesden, *Rosa anglica* (Pavia: J. A. Birreta, 1492), fol. 56r, directly inspired by Avicenna, referring to *aer corruptus in se et pestilentialis in se,* and thus being the first to cite contact (*contactum*) with lepers.

[67] *Breviarium practicae* (Lyon: A. Tardif, 1586), II.46, p. 109: *... leprosi enim inficiunt aerem et aer infectus cum attrahitur ab illis qui conversantur cum illis intrans eorum corpora inficit ea: propter hoc leprosi a conversatione sanorum hominem debent segregari... Et ideo in locis remotis habitare cogantur.*

about lepers. Also for the first time, Mondeville reflects these reservations when he writes about practitioners meeting lepers:

> No physicians or surgeons ought to bother with such cases unless they are engaged by the most intense request and at a very high price, and after their prognosis, because it is a very vile and contagious disease. Lepers like to converse with physicians and to approach them, hence the physicians who attend them, if people come to know about this, are reviled and considered as corrupted and repulsive.[68]

But if we are to believe Bernard of Gordon, this did not prevent a young bachelor in medicine, presumably better informed than others, from assiduously attending a leprous countess and even having sexual intercourse with her.[69] In 1321, during the supposed great persecution, all sorts of arguments were deployed against lepers, but none of these arguments reflects the slightest awareness of the obviously and extremely useful doctrine of contagion.[70] The first definitively to invert the perspective was Guy of Chauliac in the wake of the Black Death, which imposed a new paradigm; according to him, the main causes of leprosy are corrupted air and contact with lepers.[71] But this is a point we reach in the fourteenth century, not before. After hesitation between two pathogenic conceptions where leprosy was the consequence of either an internal struggle among confronting forces or the body's struggle against an external agent, the latter interpretation ultimately prevailed.

A survey of this evolution through medical writings imposes at least three crucial conclusions upon us. The first is the absolute impossibility of generalizing the idea of "contagiousness" and projecting an anachronistic view on the contagion of leprosy to the entire course of the Middle Ages. With regard to other sources from the early Middle Ages—Lombard legislation or Carolingian prohibitions, for example—we can concede attempts to restrict lepers during this period. These decisions may have been inspired by the paradigm of pestilence in general (readily available to the learned élite in

[68] *Chirurgia*, 424.

[69] *Lilium medicinae* XXII, p. 89–90.

[70] See M. Barber, "Lepers, Jews and Moslems: the Plot over Christendom in 1321," *History* 66 (1981): 1–17; F.-O. Touati, *Lèpre, lépreux et léproseries*, 1086–1110.

[71] Guy of Chauliac, *Chirurgia magna* (Venice: Juntas, 1546), fol. 58v (written in 1363): *Causae primitivae sunt corruptio aeris et contactus leprosorum, malitia ciborum....*

the works of classical authors) and the special attention of contemporaries to the Old Testament, but it is even more likely that they were motivated by the reality of the plague itself from the sixth to the eighth centuries, primarily in Italy.[72] But the very fact that they needed to be repeated raises the suspicion that in practice these measures were ineffective against contrary attitudes.

The second conclusion concerns the origins of the leper-houses. From the beginning of the eleventh century a real "revolution of charity" associated with dramatic economic expansion spread across the whole West, and with it the ideal of assistance, the exaltation of the poor as personifying Christ (illustrated in Great Britain by Queen Mathilda, Hugh of Lincoln, or Walter of Luci), and a wave of new foundations and aspiration to a religious life. "Brethren lepers" participated in this movement, alongside Robert of Arbrissel at Fontevraud, for example, and in leper-houses.[73] Why were such specific communities created for them? Through the sense imputed to their disease, leprosy offered a positive opportunity for redemption and sanctification. As other chronic diseases or disabilities (blindness, paralysis, ergotism, etc.) originally accepted in leper-houses (at Saint-John of Canterbury, founded by Lanfranc before 1089) or in chaplaincies (as at Gonnord near Thouarcé, to the west of Saumur, in 1087), the chronic nature of leprosy dictated against them staying in the hospitals (at Saint-Jean of Angers, at Troyes or Tournai, for example):[74] its mark in the body could be interpreted as an "opportunity" to live an experience of religious conversion more accessible and manifest than a spiritual appeal.[75] This project is reflected in the earlier organization of the communities, where lepers, identified with other monks or friars by authorities in canon law and

---

[72]Texts and references in Jeanselme, "Comment l'Europe au Moyen Age se protégea contre la lèpre," 12–13, 139–40 nos. 2–7; also F.-O. Touati, "La peste comme modèle," *Sources. Travaux historiques*, May 1990 (*Images de la maladie*), 6–8.

[73]Matthew Paris, *Chronica majora*, ed. H. R. Luard (London: Rerum britannicarum medii aevi scriptores, 1872), II, 130; *Life of St. Hugh of Lincoln*, ed. D. L. Douie and D. H. Farmer (Edinburgh: T. Nelson and Sons, 1962), II, 11–13; *Chronicon Monasterii de Bello* (London: Anglia christiana, 1846), 135; Baudri, *Vita B. Roberti de Arbrissello* (written before 1120), *PL* 162, col. 1055; Andrea, *Acta B. Roberti*, *PL* 196, col. 1073, § 33. See also F.-O. Touati, "Lèpre, sociétés, sensibilités," in *Lèpre, lépreux et léproseries*, 425–74.

[74]Rubin, *Medieval English Medicine*, 164–5; Arch. dep. Maine-et-Loire H 3178; *Statuts d'hôtels-Dieu et de léproseries*, ed. L. Le Grand (Paris: A. Picard, 1901), 25 art. 13, 115 § 90. See A. Saunier, *"Le pauvre malade" dans le cadre hospitalier médiéval: France du Nord, vers 1300–1500* (Paris: Arguments, 1993), 223.

[75]N. Beriou and F.-O. Touati, *Leprosus a Deo conversus: les lépreux entre conversion et exclusion aux XIe et XIIIe siècles* (Spoleto: Centro italiano di studi sull'Alto Medioevo, 1991; Testi, studi, strumenti, 4).

admitted to take vows, could voluntarily participate with other brothers or sisters in good health and spend the rest of their lives; it shows that it was incompatible with simple relegation.[76] Did the impact of this ideology, inspired by the greatest names of Christendom, last more than two or three generations? The growing disparity between the aptitude of most lepers, the reality of their life—formerly conceived in a wide conception of religious status, and the new exigencies of a canonical order joined to new values of the society, changed mentalities and attitudes. In social terms, from the beginning of the thirteenth century lepers became unclassifiable, and hence dangerous. The aims of leper-houses were transformed, keeping the same structures, as we see with Beaumanoir in 1283 or with the regulations of cities, as in Italy or in London at exactly the same time; beginning in 1244 at Exeter, the free access of lepers to the town was curtailed.[77]

Before the years 1230–40, perhaps earlier in southern Europe, most medical writings could offer no direct inspiration for segregative prevention. On the contrary, practitioners seem to have been ready to defend some lepers against all violent abuses or arbitrary treatment.[78] However, the penetration of new ideas and their acceptance were favoured by their confluence with social and moral considerations. The belief in sexual contamination illustrates the modalities of this process. From the fourth to the fourteenth century, a long process of sliding can be observed. For a moralist like Cesarius of Arles, leprosy served as a threat (along with other diseases, epilepsy, or infirmities) useful for moralizing, discouraging lewd behaviour, and regulating sexual

---

[76] See, for example, the major studies of A. Uyttebrouck, "Séquestration ou retraite volontaire? Quelques réflexions à propos de l'hébergement des lépreux à la léproserie de Terbank-lez-Louvain," in *Mélanges offerts à G. Jacquemyns* (Brussels: Institut de Sociologie, Université de Libre Bruxelles, 1968), 615–32; "Hôpitaux pour lépreux ou couvents de lépreux? Réflexions sur le caractère des premières grandes léproseries de nos régions à leurs origines," *Annales de la Société Belge de Histoire des Hôpitaux* 10 (1972), 5–29. See also, among other sources, Le Grand, ed., *Statuts d'hôtels-Dieu et de léproseries.*

[77] *Coutumes de Beauvaisis*, LVI, ed. A. Salmon (Paris: A. Picard, 1900), II, 326–30; J. Agrimi and C. Crisciani, *Malato, medico e medicina nel Medioevo* (Torino: Loescher, 1980), 137–8 (Bologna); D. Waley, *Les républiques médiévales italiennes* (Paris: Hachette, 1969), 109; R. M. Clay, *The Mediaeval Hospitals of England* (London: Methuen and Co., 1909), 53–5; Rubin, *Medieval English Medicine*, 158. It would be well advised to reconsider all perspectives on these restrictions, their chronology (for example, the dating of the writ *De leproso amovendo* or the rituals of separation), and the interpretations given to lepers' retreat into monasteries (as in the case of Aelfward, bishop of London, to Ramsey Abbey).

[78] For instance, John of Gaddesden, *Rosa anglica*, fol. 56r: "No one is to be adjudged a leper and isolated from all his fellows until the appearance and shape of his face be destroyed."

practices.[79] In the same sense, leprosy—as other diseases—was a common metaphor for sins like heresy. That does not mean that lepers or other sick persons were systematically seen as the incarnation of sin.[80] But at the term of this evolution, and for reasons of social necessity, this way of thinking was reversed and medical opinion itself was contaminated by connection with the new moralists' view and used for arguing the peril of all unbridled or uncontrolled sexuality. Along with prostitutes, beggars, or other vagrants, lepers were now relegated to the fringe of society and rejected as pariahs by a hostile social order.[81] The idea of air contamination, irrespective of the analogy with plague or pestilence first cited to justify it, signifies in the first instance an argument of impurity based on social intolerance, the invisible thread of rejection.

At this point one need hardly do more than state the third vital conclusion that emerges from the history of the connection between leprosy and contagion: medical writings are never autonomous, nor are they objective or neutral.

---

[79] Cesarius of Arles, *Sermo XLIV*, ed. D. G. Morin, I (Maredsous: Edition de l'abbaye, 1937), 190: ... *qui uxorem suam in profluviis positam agnoverit aut in die dominica aut in alia qualibet solemnitate adveniente se continere noluerit, qui tunc fuerint, aut leprosi, aut epileptici aut etiam forte daemoniaci nascentur....* This assertion, following Jerome, was further used in penitentials and by theologians to reprove uncontrolled sexuality.

[80] With reservations—among others—on the different levels of language and their applications: S. N. Brody, *The Disease of the Soul: Leprosy in Medieval Literature* (Ithaca: Cornell University Press, 1974), with the review by H. H. Gwin in *Cahiers de civilisation médiévale* 2 (1978): 163–5; R. I. Moore, "Heresy as Disease," in *The Concept of Heresy in the Middle Ages*, ed. W. Lourdaux and D. Verhelst (Leuven: Leuven University Press, 1983), 1–11; M. W. Bloomfield, *The Seven Deadly Sins* (Kalamazoo: Medieval Institute Publications, 1952).

[81] On the new values and social order in relation with the urbanization of society, see E. Cohen, "Le vagabondage à Paris au XIVe siècle: analyse conceptuelle," *Le Moyen Age* 88 (1982): 293–313; R. Castel, "La question sociale commence en 1349," *Cahiers de la Recherche sur le travail social* 16 (1989): 9–27; and the articles of J. Le Goff and B. Geremek in *Le travail au Moyen Age: une approche interdisciplinaire*, ed. J. Hamesse (Louvain-la-Neuve: Institut d'études médievales, 1990).

CONTRIBUTORS

Chia-Feng Chang is Assistant Professor in the Department of History, National Taiwan University. She is an executive editor of *Taiwanese Journal for the Study of Science, Technology and Medicine* and *The Newsletter for History of Chinese Science*. Her 1996 PhD dissertation was entitled *Aspects of Smallpox and Its Significance in Chinese History* (School of Oriental and African Studies, London). Her current research centres on the conceptions of *mingmen* ("gate of life") in traditional Chinese Medicine.

Lawrence I. Conrad is Historian of Near Eastern Medicine at the Wellcome Institute for the History of Medicine and President of the International Association for the Study of Traditional Asian Medicine. He has written extensively on the history of epidemic disease in the Near East, and is co-author of *The Western medical tradition: 800* BC–AD 1800 (Cambridge: Cambridge University Press, 1995). He is currently working on a history of thinking on contagion in the Islamic Near East.

Rahul Peter Das is Professor of the Philology of Modern Indian Languages at the Martin-Luther-Universität Halle-Wittenberg, Germany. Traditional Indian medicine is one of his various interests. He is co-founder and co-editor of the *Journal of the European Āyurvedic Society*. His most recent work on Indian medicine, due to appear soon, is *The Origin of the Life of a Human Being. Conception and the Female according to Ancient Indian Medical and Sexological Literature.*

Shigehisa Kuriyama is Associate Professor at the International Research Center for Japanese Studies, Kyoto, where he pursues comparative historical studies of medicine in Europe, Japan, and China. His most recent publication is *The Expressiveness of the Body and the Divergence of Greek and Chinese Medicine* (ZONE Books, 1999).

Elinor Lieber is a medical practitioner and epidemiologist and a leading authority on the history of ancient and medieval medicine, with special reference to Greek and Jewish medicine. She has worked for the World Health Organisation and at the Hadasseh Medical School, Hebrew University of Jerusalem.

Vivian Nutton is Head of the Academic Unit at the Wellcome Institute for the History of Medicine and Professor of the History of Medicine at University College London. He has written extensively on the history of medicine from Antiquity to the Renaissance, and especially on Galen. His *editio princeps* of Galen's philosophical testament *On My Own Opinions* is scheduled to appear in 1999 in the *Corpus Medicorum Graecorum* series. He contributed the sections on Antiquity and the Western Middle Ages to L.I. Conrad *et al.*, *The Western Medical Tradition, 800* BC—AD *1800* (Cambridge: Cambridge University Press, 1995), and is responsible for the medical entries in *Der neue Pauly. Enzyklopädie der Antike* (Stuttgart and Weimar: Metzler Verlag, 1996–proceeding).

François-Olivier Touati is Co-director of the Groupe de Recherches en Epistémologie et Histoire de la Médecine at the University of Paris XII, where he teaches medieval history. He is the author of two recent works on the history of leprosy: *Archives de la lèpre: atlas des léproseries entre Loire et Marne au Moyen Âge* (Paris: CTHS, 1996), and *Maladie et société an Moyen Âge: la lèpre, les lépreux et les léproseries dans la province ecclésiastique de Sens jusqu'au milieu du XIVe siècle* (Brussels: De Boeck, 1998).

Dominik Wujastyk is an Honorary Lecturer in the History of Medicine at University College, London, and Associate Curator for South Asian Collections at the Wellcome Library for the History and Understanding of Medicine. His most recent book is *The roots of Āyurveda: selections from Sanskrit medical writings* (Delhi: Penguin, 1998).

Kenneth Zysk is Associate Professor and Head of Indian Studies at Copenhagen University, where he teaches courses in Indian languages and culture. He is author of *Medicine in the Veda* (Delhi: Motilal Banarsidass, 1996) and *Asceticism and healing in ancient India. Medicine in the Buddhist monastery* (Delhi: Motilal Banarsidass, 1998). His new book, *Conjugal love in India.* Ratiśāstra *and* Ratiramaṇa. *Text, translation, and notes*, will appear shortly in the Sir Henry Wellcome Asian Series.

Index